Study Guide for

Understanding Pathophysiology

Study Guide for

Understanding Pathophysiology

Sixth Edition

Sue E. Huether, MS, PhD
Kathryn L. McCance, MS, PhD

Prepared by:

Linda Felver, PhD, RN
Associate Professor
School of Nursing
Oregon Health & Science University
Portland, Oregon

ELSEVIER

ELSEVIER

3251 Riverport Lane
St. Louis, Missouri 63043

STUDY GUIDE FOR UNDERSTANDING PATHOPHYSIOLOGY,
SIXTH EDITION

ISBN: 978-0-323-37045-5

Notices

Knowledge and best practice in this field are constantly changing. As new research and experience broaden our understanding, changes in research methods, professional practices, or medical treatment may become necessary.

Practitioners and researchers must always rely on their own experience and knowledge in evaluating and using any information, methods, compounds, or experiments described herein. In using such information or methods they should be mindful of their own safety and the safety of others, including parties for whom they have a professional responsibility.

With respect to any drug or pharmaceutical products identified, readers are advised to check the most current information provided (i) on procedures featured or (ii) by the manufacturer of each product to be administered, to verify the recommended dose or formula, the method and duration of administration, and contraindications. It is the responsibility of practitioners, relying on their own experience and knowledge of their patients, to make diagnoses, to determine dosages and the best treatment for each individual patient, and to take all appropriate safety precautions.

To the fullest extent of the law, neither the Publisher nor the authors, contributors, or editors, assume any liability for any injury and/or damage to persons or property as a matter of products liability, negligence or otherwise, or from any use or operation of any methods, products, instructions, or ideas contained in the material herein.

Executive Content Strategist: Kellie White
Content Development Manager: Luke Held
Content Development Specialist: Anna Miller
Publishing Services Manager: Hemamalini Rajendrababu
Project Manager: Maria Bernard
Designer: Margaret Reid
Cover Designer: Gopalakrishnan Venkatraman
Marketing Manager: Rebecca Ramsaroop

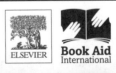

Working together
to grow libraries in
developing countries

www.elsevier.com • www.bookaid.org

Printed in United States of America

Last digit is the print number: 9 8 7 6 5 4 3 2 1

Preface

What happens in the tissues to cause the redness and swelling of inflammation? What happens in the heart during a heart attack? Why do people who have a specific disease display characteristic signs and symptoms? Learning about pathophysiology will help you answer these and other questions.

This study guide accompanies the sixth edition of *Understanding Pathophysiology* by Sue E. Huether and Kathryn L. McCance. In a logical progression, the textbook begins with the central concepts of pathophysiology at the cellular and tissue level, followed by pathophysiologic processes at the organ and system levels. This study guide follows that progression. For example, it assists with building a working knowledge of what happens in the tissues during inflammation before addressing questions regarding heart attacks and other pathophysiologies at the organ and system level.

The study guide follows the organization of the textbook, with 42 chapters. Each chapter contains a variety of activities that develop several cognitive skills, moving from the basic skills of learning definitions and acquiring knowledge to the higher-level skills of explaining, application, and integration of knowledge. Here are examples of these activities:

- **Match the Definitions:** An understanding of definitions provides the foundation for higher-level knowledge.
- **Choose the Correct Words:** Recognizing the correct word that belongs in a sentence reinforces basic knowledge acquisition.

- **Complete These Sentences:** Filling in the blanks requires more knowledge than simply recognizing words.
- **Order the Steps:** Putting the parts of a pathophysiological process into their correct sequence facilitates learning to explain them, a higher order skill.
- **Explain the Pictures:** Directed toward visual learners, these questions build explaining and integrating skills.
- **Categorize These:** Choosing the category into which items belong requires understanding them and assists with differentiating between them.
- **Describe the Difference:** These questions build the skill of comparing and contrasting, an excellent way to learn about similar items without confusing them.
- **Teach These Patients about Pathophysiology:** Unique to this study guide, these teaching activities provide the opportunity to learn pathophysiology at the level of explaining rather than rote recall.
- **Case Scenarios:** Patient examples with questions assist with application and integration of knowledge in real-world settings.

Taken together, the activities in each study guide chapter build a sequence of cognitive skills that facilitate mastery of pathophysiology at the application level needed for clinical practice.

I dedicate this study guide to my past, present, and future students.

Linda Felver

REVIEWERS

Janie Corbitt, RN, MLS
Instructor of Nursing
Retired

Kathleen Murtaugh, RN, MSN, CNA
Associate Professor
Saint Joseph's College/St. Elizabeth School of Nursing
Consortium

Linda Turchin, MSN, CNE
Associate Professor of Nursing
Fairmont State University
Fairmont, WV

Contents

1 Cellular Biology

IDENTIFY CELLULAR STRUCTURES AND THEIR FUNCTIONS

Identify the structures and match their cellular functions with their location in the picture.

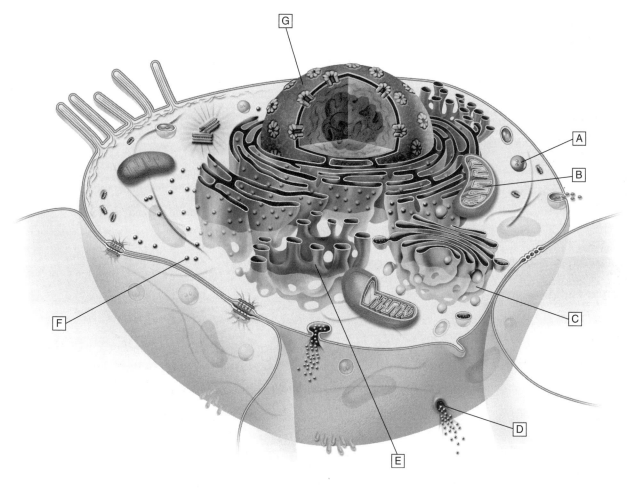

_____ 1. This structure generates ATP by oxidative phosphorylation; it is a _____.

_____ 2. This structure synthesizes proteins; it is a _____.

_____ 3. This structure processes and packages proteins for delivery; it is the _____ _____.

_____ 4. This structure serves as repository of genetic information; it is the _____.

_____ 5. This structure synthesizes and transports lipids; it is the _____ _____.

_____ 6. This structure packages and delivers proteins that are secreted; it is a secretory _____.

_____ 7. This structure contains digestive enzymes; it is a _____.

1

DESCRIBE THE DIFFERENCES

Describe the difference between each pair of terms.

8. What is the difference between a lysosome and a peroxisome?

9. What is the difference between a eukaryote and a prokaryote?

10. What is the difference between hydrophilic and hydrophobic?

MATCH THE DEFINITIONS

Match each word on the right with its definition on the left.

_____ 11. Ligand   A. Having both a hydrophobic part and a hydrophilic part

_____ 12. Amphipathic   B. Infolding of the plasma membrane to form a vesicle that enters the cell

_____ 13. Caveolae   C. The carbohydrate coating on the outer surface of the plasma membrane

_____ 14. Endocytosis   D. A substance that binds to a receptor

_____ 15. Glycocalyx   E. Tiny flask-shaped pits in the outer surface of the plasma membrane

CIRCLE THE CORRECT WORDS

Circle the correct word from the choices provided to complete these sentences.

16. The main difference between cells that divide rapidly and those that divide slowly is the amount of time they spend in the (S, G_1) phase of the cell cycle.

17. Cells develop specialized functions through the process of (differentiation, anaerobic glycolysis).

18. A particle that is dissolved is called a (substrate, solute).

19. Mitochondria need a lot of (glucose, oxygen) in order to function normally.

20. During osmosis, (particles, water molecules) move across the plasma membrane.

21. (Autocrine, Paracrine) signals act on nearby cells by (diffusion, active transport) through interstitial fluid.

22. A cell that has an insufficient oxygen supply will not be able to perform the chemistry of (the Krebs cycle, glycolysis).

23. (Active transport, Facilitated diffusion) can move substances against their concentration gradients.

24. Receptors are (proteins, lipids) that bind specific small molecules.

2

Chapter **1**   **Cellular Biology**

ORDER THE STEPS

Sequence the events that occur during each of these processes.

25. Write the letters here in the correct order of the events that occur during a neuronal action potential:

    _____

    A. Sodium ions move into the cell.
    B. Potassium ions leave the cell.
    C. Sodium permeability increases.
    D. Resting membrane potential is reestablished.
    E. Potassium permeability increases.

26. Write the letters here in the correct order of the phases of the normal cell cycle, beginning with the phase that precedes DNA synthesis: _____
    A. M phase
    B. S phase
    C. G_1 phase
    D. G_2 phase

COMPLETE THE SENTENCES

Write one word in each blank to complete these sentences.

27. Proteins in the nucleus that bind DNA and help regulate its activity are called _____.

28. Cells such as neutrophils that use hydrogen peroxide as a defensive weapon synthesize it in their _____.

29. A section of a membrane that is rich in cholesterol and helps organize membrane proteins is called a lipid _____.

30. The cells that secrete the extracellular matrix are called _____.

31. The mechanical force of water pushing against cellular membranes is called _____ pressure.

32. An _____ solution has the same osmolality as normal body fluids.

33. In a simple epithelium, the epithelial cells are in contact with a _____ membrane that provides support.

34. _____ tissue is characterized by only a few cells surrounded by a lot of extracellular matrix.

35. A myocyte is a _____ cell.

CHOOSE THE DIRECTION

For each situation, choose the direction in which the items will move. Choose A or B from the figure.

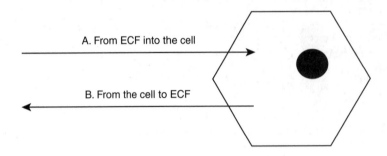

_____ 36. If the ECF becomes hypotonic, in which direction will water move?

_____ 37. If the concentration of substance X in the ECF is higher than its concentration inside the cell, in which direction will active transport move substance X?

_____ 38. If the glucose concentration in the ECF is higher than its concentration inside the cell, in which direction will facilitated diffusion move glucose?

_____ 39. In which direction does Na^+, K^+-ATPase move sodium ions?

_____ 40. In which direction does Na^+, K^+-ATPase move potassium ions?

2 Genes and Genetic Diseases

MATCH THE DEFINITIONS

Match each word on the right with its definition on the left.

_____ 1. Different version of a paired gene

_____ 2. Substance that alters genetic material (DNA)

_____ 3. Chromosome that is not a sex chromosome

_____ 4. Segment of DNA that is the basic unit of inheritance

_____ 5. Sequence of three nitrogenous bases that specifies a particular amino acid

_____ 6. Noncoding segment spliced out of mRNA

_____ 7. Alteration of DNA capable of being passed to offspring

_____ 8. Segment of mRNA that codes for proteins

_____ 9. Strand of condensed chromatin visible right before cell division

A. Codon

B. Intron

C. Exon

D. Mutation

E. Mutagen

F. Gene

G. Chromosome

H. Autosome

I. Allele

CIRCLE THE CORRECT WORDS

Circle the correct word from the choices provided to complete these sentences.

10. A somatic cell that has 46 chromosomes in its nucleus is called a (diploid cell, gamete).

11. Genetic diseases caused by (single genes, multiple genes) usually are autosomal dominant, autosomal recessive, or X-linked recessive.

12. X-linked recessive diseases are seen much more often in (females, males) than in (females, males).

13. The structure of (mRNA, DNA) is a double helix.

14. Proteins are made of a sequence of (amino acids, nucleotides).

15. If the cells have three copies of each chromosome, (triploidy, trisomy) is present.

16. (Gain, Loss) of chromosome material usually has more serious consequences than duplication of chromosome material.

17. A Barr body is an inactivated (X, Y) chromosome that is seen in normal (male, female) cells.

DESCRIBE THE DIFFERENCES

Describe the difference between each pair of terms.

18. What is the difference between heterozygous and homozygous?

19. What is the difference between monosomy and trisomy?

20. What is the difference between genotype and phenotype?

21. What is the difference between mitosis and meiosis?

ORDER THE STEPS

Sequence the events that occur during synthesis of a protein.

22. Write the letters here in the correct order of the steps: _____
    A. Translation
    B. Transcription
    C. mRNA leaves the nucleus
    D. RNA polymerase binds to DNA promoter site
    E. mRNA is spliced to remove noncoding sections

INTERPRET A PEDIGREE CHART

Examine the pedigree chart and answer the questions about it.

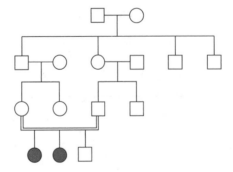

23. How many boys in this family have the genetic disorder? _____

24. What does the double line between the parents of the children with the disorder mean? _____

    _____

25. The mother of the affected children has a sister. What symbol would be used if the mother and her sister were identical twins? _____

CATEGORIZE THE CLINICAL EXAMPLES

Write the type of genetic disorder beside its clinical example. Choices: chromosomal disorder, single-gene disorder

_____ 26. Huntington disease

_____ 27. Turner syndrome

_____ 28. Down syndrome

_____ 29. Fragile X syndrome

_____ 30. Cystic fibrosis

_____ 31. Klinefelter syndrome

_____ 32. Duchenne muscular dystrophy

COMPLETE THE SENTENCES

Write one word in each blank to complete these sentences.

33. A display of chromosomes ordered according to length and centromere location is called a _____.

34. A somatic cell has _____ pairs of chromosomes.

35. A _____ mutation of DNA involves addition or deletion of a number of base pairs that is not a multiple of three and thus alters all of the codons downstream from the site of insertion or deletion.

36. A _____ gene will be expressed only if it is present in two copies.

37. People who have Down syndrome have high risk for developing _____ disease because of involvement of chromosome 21.

38. People who have the 47,XXY karyotype have _____ syndrome.

39. Interchanging of genetic material between nonhomologous chromosomes is called _____.

INTERPRET A PUNNETT SQUARE

Examine the Punnett square and determine what mode of inheritance it depicts.

Normal parent

		d	d
Affected parent	D	Dd Heterozygous affected	Dd Heterozygous affected
	d	dd Homozygous normal	dd Homozygous normal

40. This Punnett square represents what type of genetic condition?
    A. Autosomal dominant
    B. Autosomal recessive with two heterozygous carriers
    C. X-linked recessive with normal male and female carrier

TEACH PEOPLE ABOUT PATHOPHYSIOLOGY

Write your response to each situation in the space provided.

41. Mr. and Mrs. Medlow's infant Kira has phenylketonuria (PKU), an autosomal recessive disorder. "Tell me how Kira could inherit PKU from us when neither of us has it," says Mr. Medlow. "I remember what genes are, but if we both have the PKU gene, why don't we have the disease like Kira does?"

42. "What does *autosomal* mean?" asks Mr. Medlow.

43. "I know a child who has cystic fibrosis," says Mrs. Medlow. "That is genetic too, isn't it?"

44. "If cystic fibrosis is autosomal recessive like PKU, why can't they manage it by diet like we do for Kira's PKU?" says Mrs. Medlow.

3 Epigenetics and Disease

MATCH THE DEFINITIONS

Match each word on the right with its definition on the left.

_____ 1. Protein around which DNA winds   A. Transcription

_____ 2. Process of making mRNA from a section of DNA   B. Chromatin

_____ 3. Proteins and DNA in the nucleus   C. Gene

_____ 4. Section of DNA that carries the code for a protein or noncoding RNA   D. Histone

CIRCLE THE CORRECT WORDS

Circle the correct word from the choices provided to complete these sentences.

5. Epigenetics is regulation of gene expression (caused by, not caused by) altered DNA sequence.

6. DNA methylation leads to (activation, silencing) of genes.

7. Epigenetic modifications (are, are not) maintained in successive mitotic cell divisions.

8. The process of predictable gene silencing on one copy of a chromosome but not on the other, depending on which parent transmits the chromosome, is known as (imprinting, epigenetics).

9. (miRNA, mRNA) carries the code for a protein to a ribosome, but (miRNA, mRNA) can regulate gene expression.

10. In contrast to DNA sequence mutations, which (can, cannot) be altered directly, some epigenetic modifications (can, cannot) be reversed.

11. Studies of (cousins, twins) are used to investigate epigenetic modifications over time.

DESCRIBE THE DIFFERENCES

Describe the difference between each pair of terms.

12. What is the difference between mRNA and ncRNA?

13. What is the difference between histones and chromatin?

14. What is the difference between euchromatin and heterochromatin?

COMPLETE THE SENTENCES

Write one word in each blank to complete these sentences.

15. Overactivity of insulin-like growth factor 2 (IGF-2) causes overgrowth in _____ syndrome, but down-regulation of IGF-2 causes the diminished growth seen in _____ syndrome.

16. A gene that has methylation in its _____ region is less likely to be transcribed into mRNA.

17. MicroRNAs that stimulate development and progression of cancer are called _____.

18. Genes that are necessary to maintain function of all types of cells and normally remain transcriptionally active are called _____ genes.

19. Hereditary transmission of epigenetic changes to successive generations is called _____ _____.

20. Environmental chemicals, dietary factors, and alcohol intake can modify gene expression by causing _____ modifications.

IDENTIFY THE ENZYMES

Write the name of the enzymes in the blanks. Choices: histone acetylases; DNA methyltransferases; histone deacetylases

21. Add acetyl groups to histone tails: _____

22. Remove acetyl groups from histone tails: _____

23. Attach methyl groups to nucleotides in DNA: _____

TEACH PEOPLE ABOUT PATHOPHYSIOLOGY

Write your response to each situation in the space provided.

24. "I am reading a journal article about cancer development," says another nurse. "What happens when the promoter region of tumor suppressor genes is hypermethylated? Does that encourage or discourage development of cancer?"

25. "What is noncoding RNA?" says Mr. Stevens. "When I studied biology in college, we learned about the genetic code and RNA, but I do not understand what noncoding RNA would be. Please explain."

26. "How is it possible for several types of cells to arise from one kind of stem cell?" asks a medical student. "I know that all cells have the same DNA, but different genes are active in different cell types. Help me understand."

CLINICAL SCENARIO

Read the clinical scenario and answer the questions to explore your understanding of genomic imprinting.

Robbie Taylor, age 4, who has Prader-Willi syndrome, has come for a well-child examination. No symptoms have been reported by parents or child. Moderate mental developmental delay has been verified by a psychologist.

Physical Examination

- Vital signs normal

- Muscle tone diminished

- Height below normal for age; BMI in obesity range

- Hands and feet appear small in relation to body size

- Genitals underdeveloped for age

27. What causes Prader-Willi syndrome?

28. In Prader-Willi syndrome, which copy of the crucial genes is imprinted?

29. Does imprinting of these genes occur normally, or is this an abnormal occurrence?

30. How is it possible for Prader-Willi syndrome and Angelman syndrome to arise from a defect in the same location of the same chromosome?

4 Altered Cellular and Tissue Biology

MATCH THE DEFINITIONS

Match each word on the right with its definition on the left.

_____ 1. Stiffening of skeletal muscles after death

_____ 2. Area of cell death in which cells are digested by their own enzymes, becoming soft and runny

_____ 3. A type of cellular housekeeping in which a cell digests some of its own components

_____ 4. Area of cell death in which dead cells disintegrate, but the debris is not digested completely by enzymes

_____ 5. Area of cell death in which denatured proteins appear firm and opaque

_____ 6. An atom or group of atoms having an unpaired electron

_____ 7. Purple discoloration of dependent tissues after death

_____ 8. Cell death that involves orderly dismantling of cell components and packaging the remainders in vesicles

A. Apoptosis

B. Free radical

C. Livor mortis

D. Liquefactive necrosis

E. Rigor mortis

F. Coagulative necrosis

G. Autophagy

H. Caseous necrosis

CATEGORIZE THE CLINICAL EXAMPLES

Write the type of cellular adaptation beside its clinical example. Choices: atrophy, hypertrophy, hyperplasia, metaplasia.

_____ 9. Lining of uterus thickens after ovulation because of increased amounts of estrogen.

_____ 10. Man who lifts weights regularly develops larger biceps.

_____ 11. Thymus gland decreases in size during childhood.

_____ 12. Columnar epithelium in bronchi of cigarette smoker is replaced by stratified squamous epithelium.

_____ 13. Captain of roller derby team has greater thigh diameter on left than right from skating clockwise.

_____ 14. Left calf is smaller than right calf when cast is removed from it.

_____ 15. Liver regenerates after surgical removal of damaged portion.

CIRCLE THE CORRECT WORDS

Circle the correct word from the choices provided to complete these sentences.

16. Cell death by (necrosis, apoptosis) causes inflammation, but cell death by (necrosis, apoptosis) does not.

17. Dysplasia also is called (normal, atypical) hyperplasia.

18. Release of (potassium, calcium) ions from intracellular stores into the cytoplasm during ischemia damages the cell.

19. Compared with normal aerobic metabolism, cells that use anaerobic metabolism produce (more, less) ATP and (more, less) lactic acid.

20. The most important way to prevent medication-related poisoning deaths in children is safe (storage, prescribing) of medications.

21. Reactive oxygen species, such as (superoxide radicals, superoxide dismutase) damage cells by attacking their (potassium, membranes).

22. Postmortem changes (involve, do not involve) the inflammatory response.

23. Gangrene occurs when cells die of (hypoxia, trauma) and (poisoning, bacterial invasion).

ORDER THE STEPS

Beginning with the acute obstruction of a coronary artery, sequence the events that occur during necrosis of a myocardial cell.

24. Write the letters here in the correct order of the steps: _____
    A. ATP supply decreases within the cell.
    B. Acute obstruction of coronary artery cuts off arterial blood supply to myocardium.
    C. Cell runs on anaerobic metabolism because of lack of oxygen.
    D. Cell bursts and spills its contents into the interstitial fluid.
    E. Active transport of ions across the cell membrane slows.
    F. Lysosomal enzymes destroy components of their own cell.
    G. Osmosis causes cell swelling, and calcium accumulates in the cell.
    H. Organelles, including lysosomes, swell and rupture.

DESCRIBE THE DIFFERENCES

Describe the difference between each pair of terms.

25. What is the difference between hypertrophy and hyperplasia?

26. What is the difference between suffocation and strangulation?

27. What is the difference between an abrasion and a laceration?

28. What is the difference between dystrophic calcification and metastatic calcification?

29. What is the difference between a penetrating gunshot wound and a perforating gunshot wound?

COMPLETE THE SENTENCES

Write one word in each blank to complete these sentences.

30. Acute cellular swelling during ischemia is reversible if _____ is supplied quickly.

31. Active tuberculosis is characterized by _____ necrosis, whereas death of brain cells is characterized by _____ necrosis.

32. During apoptosis, cell contents are contained in vesicles called _____ _____, which are removed by _____.

33. Liver enzymes metabolize most blood ethanol to _____, which damages tissues.

34. When excessive reactive oxygen species overwhelm the endogenous antioxidant systems, _____ _____ occurs.

35. Death of the entire person is called _____ death.

36. Melanin is synthesized by epidermal cells called _____ and accumulates in other epidermal cells called _____.

37. Active enzymes that dismantle the cellular components during apoptosis are called _____.

RESPOND TO THESE CLINICAL SITUATIONS

Place yourself in these situations and write your responses in the spaces provided.

38. Mr. Martin had severe crushing injuries of both lower extremities when his house collapsed on him during an earthquake. Among other abnormal values, his laboratory tests show elevated creatine kinase in his blood. Why is his blood creatine kinase high?

39. Mrs. Santosa died peacefully in her sleep at home while lying prone. When her relatives discovered her body and rolled her over, they saw purple discoloration of half of her face and of her abdomen. They are very concerned that she might have been beaten the night before she died. What factual information do they need to relieve their concern?

Chapter **4 Altered Cellular and Tissue Biology**

40. The entire Berg family was in the hospital room when Mrs. Berg died quietly from terminal cancer. As the family is preparing to leave, Kevin Berg, age 10, says to his mother, "I think grandma is not really dead. She is just sleeping. Dead people are stiff as boards. I saw that on TV. Grandma's hands are cold, but her arms are not stiff." His mother looks at the nurse for help. In addition to addressing the emotional issues, what factual information should be provided?

DRAW YOUR ANSWERS

Read the questions and draw your answers.

These are normal cells that are capable of cell division and normally receive basal levels of hormonal stimulation.

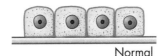

Normal

41. Draw what these cells would look like after their hormonal stimulation has been reduced substantially for several weeks.

42. Draw what these cells would look like after receiving excessive hormonal stimulation for several weeks.

IDENTIFY THE CHARACTERISTICS

Choose the characteristic(s) of apoptosis. You may select more than one answer. Choose all that apply.

43. Write the letters of your choice(s) here: _____
    A. Cell is damaged by its own lysosomal enzymes.
    B. Cell shrinks when its cytoskeleton is dismantled.
    C. Cell injury is reversible if nutrients are restored in time.
    D. Process causes inflammation.
    E. Sections of the cell bud off into vesicles.
    F. Cell swells when osmosis occurs.
    G. Process occurs when caspases are inactivated.

TEACH PEOPLE ABOUT PATHOPHYSIOLOGY

Write your response to each situation in the space provided.

44. Kenesha Francis, age 9, broke her arm 6 weeks ago, and the cast will be removed today. Before the cast is removed, teach her about the expected appearance of her arm in words appropriate to her age.

45. "The doctor said my heart enlarged because my blood pressure is high," says Mr. Hendricks. "Please explain that!"

46. Mr. Lapin has diabetes and will have amputation of the toes shown in the photograph.

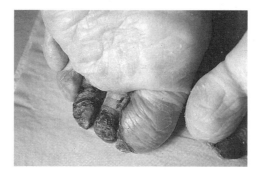

He says, "Why did my toes get black and hard rather than swollen and mushy like my Dad's toes did before surgery?"

5 Fluids and Electrolytes, Acids and Bases

MATCH THE DEFINITIONS

Match each word on the right with its definition on the left.

_____ 1. Excessive carbon dioxide in the blood

_____ 2. Excessive sodium concentration in the blood

_____ 3. Fluid accumulation in interstitial spaces

_____ 4. Fluid accumulation in the peritoneal cavity

_____ 5. Decreased pH of the blood

_____ 6. Excessive potassium concentration in the blood

A. Edema

B. Ascites

C. Acidosis

D. Hypercapnia

E. Hyperkalemia

F. Hypernatremia

CIRCLE THE CORRECT WORDS

Circle the correct word from the choices provided to complete these sentences.

7. The osmolality of the intracellular fluid normally is (higher than, the same as, lower than) the extracellular fluid because water crosses cell membranes (with difficulty, freely) through aquaporins.

8. (Sodium, Albumin) is primarily responsible for the plasma oncotic pressure.

9. Thirst prompts fluid intake through action of (baroreceptors, osmoreceptors) located in the (hypothalamus, posterior pituitary).

10. Isotonic fluid excess causes (hypernatremia, hypervolemia).

11. Renal compensation for an acid-base balance is (fast, slow); pulmonary compensation for an acid-base balance is (fast, slow).

12. Fluid moves out of capillaries by (osmosis, filtration) and into or out of cells by (osmosis, filtration).

13. Hypercapnia means an excess of (metabolic acid, carbon dioxide) in the blood.

14. The most dangerous effect of hyperkalemia is its action on the (kidneys, heart).

CATEGORIZE THE CAUSES OF EDEMA

Write the major cause of the edema beside each clinical situation. Choices: increased capillary hydrostatic pressure, decreased plasma oncotic pressure, increased capillary permeability, lymphatic obstruction.

_____ 15. Tumor grows in lymph node

_____ 16. Right heart failure

_____ 17. Infected wound

_____ 18. Clot in a vein

_____ 19. Protein malnutrition

_____ 20. Bee sting

_____ 21. End-stage renal disease

SELECT THE GREATER

Consider the pairs and select the one that is greater.

22. Who has a greater percentage of body weight as water: a lean woman or an obese woman?

23. Who has a greater percentage of body weight as water: an infant or an adult?

24. Who has a greater percentage of body weight as water, if both people weigh the same: a woman or a man?

25. Who has a greater percentage of body weight as water, if both people weigh the same: a 56-year-old man or a 78-year-old man?

26. Where is the potassium ion concentration greater: extracellular fluid or intracellular fluid?

27. Where is the sodium ion concentration greater: extracellular fluid or intracellular fluid?

28. Which is greater: the pH of an acid solution or the pH of an alkaline solution?

29. Which is greater: the respiratory rate during metabolic acidosis or the respiratory rate during metabolic alkalosis?

EXPLAIN THE PICTURES

Examine the pictures and answer the questions about them.

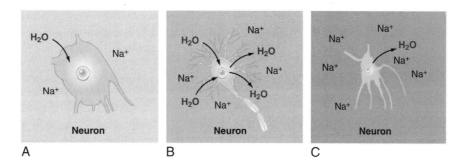

A   B   C

30. Compare the sodium concentration in panels A and B. Panel B shows isotonic fluid, so the fluid in A is _____ and the fluid in C is _____.

31. Why did the neuron in panel A swell?

32. What cerebral clinical manifestations occur when neurons swell as in panel A?

33. Why are the cerebral clinical manifestations of the situation in panel C very similar to those in panel A?

Chapter **5 Fluids and Electrolytes, Acids and Bases**

CHARACTERIZE THE HORMONES

Write one letter and one number by each hormone in the left column to indicate the stimuli that increase its secretion and its physiologic effects when secreted.

Hormone	Choose the Stimuli That Increase Secretion of the Hormone	Choose the Physiologic Effects of the Hormone
_____ 34. Aldosterone	A. High plasma calcium	1. Increases renal sodium and water excretion
_____ 35. Parathyroid hormone	B. Increased plasma osmolality, substantially decreased arterial blood pressure	2. Increases renal sodium and water reabsorption; increases renal excretion of potassium and hydrogen ions
_____ 36. Atrial natriuretic peptide	C. Low plasma calcium	3. Increases resorption of bone; stimulates renal reabsorption of calcium; inhibits renal reabsorption of phosphate
_____ 37. Calcitonin	D. Increased volume in the cardiac atria	4. Increases renal water reabsorption, vasoconstriction
_____ 38. Antidiuretic hormone	E. Angiotensin II, increased plasma potassium	5. Inhibits osteoclasts in bone

DESCRIBE THE DIFFERENCES

Describe the difference between each pair of terms.

39. What is the difference between interstitial fluid and extracellular fluid?

40. What is the difference between a volatile acid and a nonvolatile acid?

41. What is the difference between acidemia and acidosis?

42. With regard to an acid-base imbalance, what is the difference between correction and compensation?

COMPLETE THE SENTENCES

Write one word in each blank to complete these sentences.

43. One third of body water is in the _____ fluid, and two thirds is in the _____ fluid.

44. A standard 70-kg man has approximately _____ liters of total body water.

45. Excessive fluid within the interstitial space is called _____.

46. An _____ fluid has the same concentration of solute as the plasma.

47. A person who has a lung disease may develop a primary _____ acid-base imbalance, but a person who has a kidney disease may develop a primary _____ acid-base imbalance.

48. When the blood pH is 7.40, the bicarbonate-to-carbonic acid ratio is _____.

49. The two most important plasma buffers are _____ and _____.

50. Calculating the anion gap may help to distinguish between different causes of metabolic _____.

51. Overuse of phosphate-containing over-the-counter enemas can cause _____, which in turn will _____ the plasma calcium concentration.

ASSESS THE PATIENTS

Write one letter and one number by each patient situation in the left column to indicate the imbalance(s) for which that patient has high risk and the assessment findings for the imbalance(s).

Patient	Choose the Imbalance(s) for Which the Patient Has High Risk	Choose the Assessment Findings That Indicate the High-Risk Imbalance(s)
_____ 52. Mrs. Singh takes glucocorticoids for a chronic disease.	A. Isotonic fluid deficit, hypokalemia, metabolic alkalosis	1. Paresthesias of fingers, lightheadedness, confusion
_____ 53. Mr. Wiggins has been sobbing and breathing deeply and rapidly for an hour since his wife died.	B. Isotonic fluid excess and hypokalemia	2. Slow shallow respirations, blood pH less than 7.35, blood $PaCO_2$ increased
_____ 54. Mr. Jenkins is comatose from a heroin overdose.	C. Hypercalcemia	3. Dependent edema, weight gain, distended neck veins when upright, skeletal muscle weakness, constipation, abdominal distention
_____ 55. Baby Thompson has repeated vomiting from pyloric stenosis.	D. Respiratory acidosis	4. Fatigue, weakness, anorexia, constipation, lethargy
_____ 56. Mrs. Smythe has hyperparathyroidism.	E. Respiratory alkalosis	5. Tachycardia; rapid weight loss; decreased urine output; skeletal muscle weakness; slow, shallow respirations; lethargy

CHOOSE THE DIRECTION

For each situation, choose the direction in which the items will move. Choose A or B from the figure.

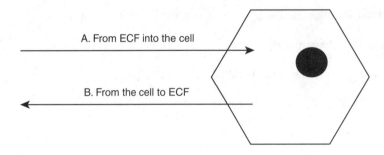

A. From ECF into the cell

B. From the cell to ECF

_____ 57. In which direction does insulin move potassium ions?

_____ 58. In which direction does epinephrine move potassium ions?

_____ 59. In which direction does alkalosis move potassium ions?

_____ 60. In which direction does hypernatremia move water?

TEACH PEOPLE ABOUT PATHOPHYSIOLOGY

Write your response to each situation in the space provided.

61. Mr. Sheehan has bilateral ankle edema from congestive heart failure. "Are my ankles inflamed?" he says. "I know that inflammation causes swelling."

62. Mrs. Kiley, who is taking care of her husband at home after his hospitalization for a stroke, was told to call the doctor if Mr. Kiley develops dependent edema. She says, "I know what edema looks like, but where is dependent edema located?"

63. Mr. Janus, who is having his first renal dialysis session, says, "I know that my failed kidneys cannot excrete acids, but I did not eat any acids, so why did I get metabolic acidosis?"

64. Ms. Winsom, age 16, has diabetic ketoacidosis. "Why is she breathing so fast?" says her father. "Does she have pneumonia as well as diabetes ketoacidosis?"

65. "Tell me the most common fluid, electrolyte, and acid-base imbalances in oliguric end-stage renal disease patients," says a nurse. "I am being sent to help on the renal unit this morning."

CLINICAL SCENARIO

Read the clinical scenario and answer the questions to explore your understanding of fluid, electrolyte, and acid-base imbalances.

Mrs. Tanaka, age 76, was brought to an urgent care facility because she fell when she stood up after sitting all afternoon in her apartment where she lives alone. Although slow to answer questions, Mrs. Tanaka states she has muscle weakness, muscle cramping, and constipation. She has had diarrhea for 3 weeks. Physical examination with Mrs. Tanaka supine revealed flat neck veins, HR 102 beats/min, pulse regular but weak, BP 90/56 mm Hg, respirations 20 breaths/min and deep. The on-site clinical laboratory provided these results: serum sodium 142 mEq/L, potassium 2.8 mEq/L.

66. What fluid imbalance does Mrs. Tanaka have? _____ What data support that?

67. What imbalance is indicated by her laboratory results? _____ What other clinical manifestations are consistent with that imbalance?

68. What additional electrolyte imbalance(s) might Mrs. Tanaka have? Provide supporting data.

69. Mrs. Tanaka may have an acid-base imbalance. Which one? _____ What aspects of her history and clinical presentation support that?

70. Mrs. Tanaka was given intravenous isotonic sodium chloride, with appropriate electrolyte in it. What was the purpose of administering that particular fluid?

6 Innate Immunity: Inflammation and Wound Healing

MATCH THE DEFINITIONS

Match each word on the right with its definition on the left.

_____ 1. A signaling molecule that attracts white blood cells

_____ 2. A pattern recognition protein on innate immune cells

_____ 3. Substance released by damaged cells that activates coagulation

_____ 4. Enzyme that degrades fibrin polymers in clots

A. Toll-like receptor

B. Tissue factor

C. Plasmin

D. Chemokine

MATCH THE FUNCTIONS

Match the functions on the right with the cells on the left.

_____ 5. Eosinophils

_____ 6. Mast cells

_____ 7. Natural killer cells

_____ 8. Macrophages

_____ 9. Neutrophils

A. Eliminate virus-infected cells

B. Phagocytize microorganisms and cellular debris; secrete chemicals that promote tissue healing; activate adaptive immunity

C. Defend against parasites; degrade vasoactive substances released by mast cells

D. Phagocytize microorganisms and cellular debris soon after injury; secrete chemicals that call in longer-acting phagocytes

E. Release chemicals that initiate the inflammatory response

CIRCLE THE CORRECT WORDS

Circle the correct words from the choices provided to complete these sentences.

10. The first line of defense against microorganisms is (anatomic barriers, phagocytic cells).

11. Surfactant and other chemical defenses produced by lung epithelium are called (collectins, resistin-like molecules).

12. The microorganisms that normally colonize the body surfaces are called the normal (microbiome, bacteriocins).

13. (Kinins, Defensins) are antimicrobial peptides, but (kinins, defensins) are proteins that become activated in the inflammatory response.

14. One innate immune cell can recognize many different types of pathogenic bacteria because it has (pattern recognition receptors, adhesion molecules).

15. A membrane attack complex, formed by the activated (complement, coagulation) cascade, causes (clot formation, cell lysis).

COMPLETE THE OVERVIEW TABLE

Complete this table by writing the correct letter in each blank in the table.
- A. T and B lymphocytes, antibodies
- B. Skin, mucous membranes, gastric acid, microbiome
- C. Phagocytes and some nonphagocytic immune cells, inflammatory response

Nonspecific Defense Mechanisms		Specific Defense Mechanisms
First Line of Defense: Closed Barrier	Second Line of Defense: Innate Immunity	Third Line of Defense: Adaptive (Acquired) Immunity
16. _____	17. _____	18. _____

CATEGORIZE THE IMMUNE CELLS

Write the type of immune cell beside its name. Choices: phagocytic innate, nonphagocytic innate, adaptive.

_____ 19. Mast cell

_____ 20. Lymphocyte

_____ 21. Macrophage

_____ 22. Neutrophil

ORDER THE STEPS

Sequence the events that occur during acute inflammation.

23. Write the letters here in the correct order of the steps: _____
- A. Local edema
- B. Tissue damage caused by injury
- C. Increased vascular permeability
- D. Leakage of plasma into tissues
- E. Vasodilation
- F. White blood cell margination and entry into tissues

Sequence the events that occur when a circulating neutrophil enters tissue and phagocytizes a microorganism.

24. Write the letters here in the correct order of the steps: _____
- A. Diapedesis
- B. Engulfment and formation of phagosome
- C. Margination
- D. Recognition and attachment
- E. Formation of phagolysosome
- F. Destruction of the microorganism
- G. Increased adhesion molecules
- H. Chemotaxis

DESCRIBE THE DIFFERENCES

Describe the difference between each pair of terms.

25. What is the difference between a PAMP and a DAMP?

26. What is the difference between opsonins and cytokines?

EXPLAIN THE PICTURES

Examine the pictures and answer the questions about them.

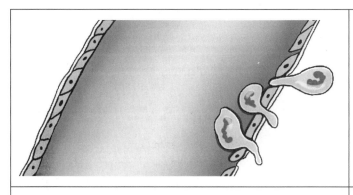

27. What one word describes what these cells are doing? _____

28. After these cells have left the blood vessel, what directs them to the site of tissue injury?

29. What does *PMN* mean? _____

30. Which cell is the PMN? _____

 A   B

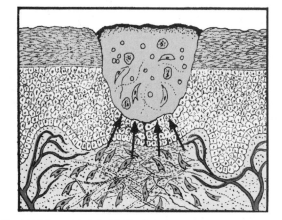

31. In this picture of a healing wound, fibroblasts are migrating into the area. Which phagocytic cells secrete chemicals to attract them? _____

_____

32. What is the function of these fibroblasts?

33. Does wound contraction occur before or after fibroblast migration and proliferation? _____

_____

Chapter **6** **Innate Immunity: Inflammation and Wound Healing**

COMPLETE THE SENTENCES

Write one word in each blank to complete these sentences.

34. *Natural immunity* and *native immunity* are other terms for _____ immunity.

35. During chronic inflammation, the body may wall off an infectious agent by forming a _____.

36. Plasma protein systems such as complement are called _____ because each component of the system activates the next component.

37. A raised scar that extends beyond the original boundaries of the wound is called a _____.

38. Wound _____ is the pulling apart of a wound at the suture line.

39. Activated mast cells release _____ inflammatory mediators immediately and release other inflammatory mediators more slowly after _____ them.

CHARACTERIZE THE EXUDATES

Match the characteristics on the right with the types of exudates on the left.

_____ 40. Fibrinous exudate   A. Watery, with few proteins or cells

_____ 41. Purulent exudate   B. Another term for purulent exudate

_____ 42. Hemorrhagic exudate   C. Thick and clotted

_____ 43. Suppurative exudate   D. Containing many red blood cells

_____ 44. Serous exudate   E. Containing many white blood cells

APPLY KNOWLEDGE IN CLINICAL SITUATIONS

Apply your knowledge by choosing the best answer for each question in these clinical situations.

45. Mr. Mewe lay on a concrete floor for 9 hours after a heroin overdose and developed a deep pressure sore on his sacrum. He was taken to drug rehab, and his wound is healing with no complications. Which term should a nurse use when describing this mode of healing to a professional colleague?
    A. Callus formation
    B. Primary intention
    C. Remodeling
    D. Secondary intention

46. Emily, age 6, has an infected finger and has just been given an antibiotic. Her mother is very worried because the finger is red and swollen. After a nurse tells her that these signs will go away as the infection and inflammation resolve, Emily's mother says, "Isn't inflammation really bad for you? It feels so bad." She needs to know that acute inflammation:
    A. causes serious delays in wound healing.
    B. results in pain and tissue destruction.
    C. promotes the spread of bacteria to the other tissue.
    D. neutralizes and destroys microorganisms.

47. A new nurse says, "Why is fever associated with inflammation? What causes it?" Choose the best response.
    A. Inflammatory chemicals called cytokines cause fever.
    B. Mast cell degranulation causes fever.
    C. Infection causes fever, especially bacterial infection.
    D. Macrophage chemotaxis causes fever.

48. Mrs. Tuttle had a hysterectomy 2 days ago. A nurse who is doing discharge teaching is discussing the importance of rest and nutrition when Mrs. Tuttle interrupts. "I can take pain pills if it hurts," she says. "I am a very busy person and do not have time to rest!" What principle should underlie the nurse's response?
   A. Inflammation is a necessary component of wound healing.
   B. Wound contraction takes time, and rest and good nutrition will assist it.
   C. Reconstruction and maturation enable a healing wound to be strong.
   D. When epithelialization has occurred, tissue healing is nearly complete.

49. Mrs. Kienow has inflamed knuckles from rheumatoid arthritis. "Why do my poor inflamed finger joints feel so hot when I touch them?" she asks. Choose the best response.
   A. More warm blood comes to the inflamed area.
   B. Heat means that your small blood vessels are leaky.
   C. Infecting bacteria produce heat by fast metabolism.
   D. Invading immune cells from your blood cause the heat.

TEACH PEOPLE ABOUT PHYSIOLOGY

Write your response to each situation in the space provided.

50. "What is innate immunity?" says Mr. Birde. "I thought you have to be vaccinated to get immunity."

51. "Why is my knee so red?" says Jessica, age 7, who scraped her knee when she fell on the playground. "I want to know why!"

52. "I understand why it hurts, but what makes a sprained ankle swell up like that?" asks Mrs. Kellerman.

53. "How do my white blood cells know how to get to this infected mosquito bite?" says David, age 14. "I thought white blood cells are in the blood."

54. "That nurse said that healing this ulcer is only her secondary intention," says Mr. Dow, who has a sacral pressure ulcer. "That is ridiculous! This pressure ulcer is the reason that I am here!"

55. "My doctor said I got this fungus because penicillin killed off my normal microbiome," says Mrs. Hunt. "What does 'normal microbiome' mean?"

7 Adaptive Immunity

MATCH THE DEFINITIONS

Match the word on the right with its definition on the left.

_____ 1. Antibody-producing cell

_____ 2. Cell that suppresses immune response to self-antigens

_____ 3. Small antigen that binds to large molecules and induces an immune
response

_____ 4. Portion of an antigen that is recognized by an antibody or specific
lymphocyte receptor

_____ 5. Molecule that activates many Th2 cell receptors regardless of their antigen
specificity by binding in an unusual location

A. Hapten

B. Superantigen

C. Epitope

D. Plasma cell

E. T-regulatory cell

COMPLETE THE OVERVIEW

Fill in the two blanks to complete the overview of immunity.

6.

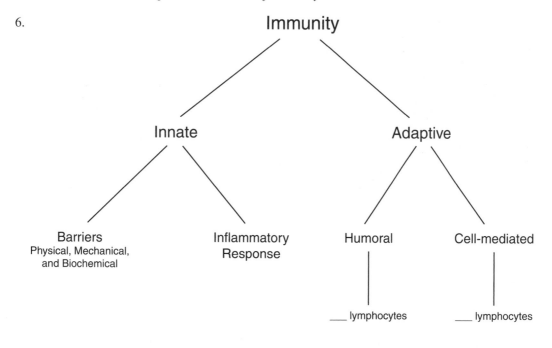

Immunity

- Innate
  - Barriers
    Physical, Mechanical,
    and Biochemical
  - Inflammatory
    Response
- Adaptive
  - Humoral
    ___ lymphocytes
  - Cell-mediated
    ___ lymphocytes

CIRCLE THE CORRECT WORDS

Circle the correct words from the choices provided to complete these sentences.

7. Human MHC molecules are known as (APC, HLA) antigens.

8. MHC class I molecules present (exogenous, endogenous) antigens, whereas MHC class II molecules present (exogenous, endogenous) antigens.

9. (Dendritic cells, Neutrophils) are the most effective in presenting antigen to naive immunocompetent Th cells.

10. Physical interactions between B lymphocytes and (Th1, Th2) cells usually are necessary for B lymphocytes to become activated.

CATEGORIZE THE CLINICAL EXAMPLES

Write the type of immunity beside each clinical example. Choices: active, passive.

_____ 11. Neonate does not develop an infection because he has maternal antibodies that he received in breast milk.

_____ 12. Child does not develop an infection because she has been immunized against it.

_____ 13. Man does not develop an infection because he was infected with that same microorganism previously and recovered.

_____ 14. Woman does not develop an infection because she was given gamma globulin after being exposed to an infected person.

ORDER THE STEPS

Sequence the events that occur during development of a mature CD4+ cell.

15. Write the letters here in the correct order of the steps: _____
    A. APC presents processed antigen with MHC class II molecules to T cell.
    B. Lymphoid stem cell migrates to thymus.
    C. T cell differentiates and matures to CD4+ cell.
    D. Cell divides and differentiates, developing T-cell receptors and surface markers.
    E. Immunocompetent naive T cell migrates to secondary lymphoid organ.

DESCRIBE THE DIFFERENCES

Describe the difference between each pair of terms.

16. What is the difference between central and peripheral tolerance?

17. What is the difference between the targets of antibodies and cytotoxic T cells?

18. What is the difference between the location of MHC class I molecules and MHC class II molecules?

EXPLAIN THE PICTURES

Examine the pictures and answer the questions about them.

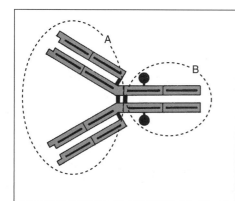

19. Which circle shows the Fab fragment of this Ig? _____

20. Why is the Fab fragment important?

21. Which circle shows the Fc fragment? _____

22. In what way is it beneficial that some innate immune cells have Fc receptors?

23. Look at the labels on the graph. Does this graph pertain to the innate immune system or the adaptive immune system?

24. Which curves rise sooner after exposure to antigen, those in section A or section B? _____

25. Why do the curves you identified rise sooner after antigen exposure?

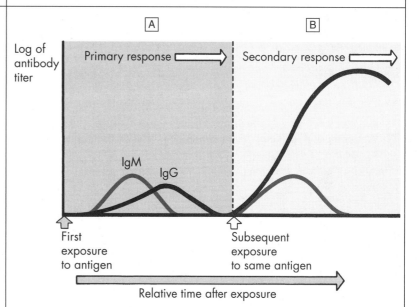

CHARACTERIZE THE IMMUNOGLOBULINS

Match the characteristics on the right with the types of immunoglobulins on the left.

_____ 26. IgE   A. Most abundant class of Igs; are transported across the placenta

_____ 27. IgM   B. Low concentration in blood; are surface receptors on developing B lymphocytes

_____ 28. IgG   C. Active against parasites; are important mediators of allergic responses

_____ 29. IgA   D. Produced during the primary response to antigen; are the largest Igs

_____ 30. IgD   E. Most abundant in body secretions

COMPLETE THE SENTENCES

Write one word in each blank to complete these sentences.

31. Another name for antigenic determinant is _____.

32. CD1 antigen-presenting molecules present exogenous _____ antigens.

33. Helper T cells are MHC class _____ restricted, but cytotoxic T cells are MHC class _____ restricted.

34. The secondary immune response also is called the _____ response.

35. Cytokines secreted by Th1 cells promote _____ immunity; cytokines secreted by Th2 cells promote _____ immunity; cytokines secreted by Th17 cells activate _____; cytokines secreted by Treg cells _____ the immune response.

36. The term *class-switch* indicates that a B lymphocyte changes from producing _____ to producing another class of immunoglobulin.

TEACH PEOPLE ABOUT PHYSIOLOGY

Write your response to each situation in the space provided.

37. A nurse tells Jason, age 14, that he will make antibodies after his immunization. "What good are antibodies, anyway?" asks Jason.

38. "Antibodies are proteins," says Nurse Lee. "How can infants get antibodies through breast milk? Wouldn't they be digested?"

39. "The medical student said that NK cells are my friends when I have a virus infection," says Mrs. Collins. "What are NK cells? Are they the ones that make antibodies?"

8 Infection and Defects in Mechanisms of Defense

MATCH THE DEFINITIONS

Match each word on the right with its definition on the left.

_____ 1. Ability to spread from one individual to others and cause disease

A. Virulence

_____ 2. Immune system of one individual produces an immunologic reaction against tissues of another individual

B. Communicability

_____ 3. Capacity of an organism to cause severe disease

C. Opportunistic

_____ 4. Normally not causing disease, but able to do so when an individual's immune system is suppressed

D. Alloimmunity

_____ 5. Altered immunologic response to an antigen that results in disease or damage to the host

E. Allergy

_____ 6. Deleterious effects of immunologic response to environmental antigens

F. Hypersensitivity

CATEGORIZE THE ORGANISMS

Write the type of organism beside its name. Choices: bacterium, virus, fungus, parasite.

_____ 7. *Aspergillus*

_____ 8. *Staphylococcus*

_____ 9. *Candida*

_____ 10. *Plasmodium*

_____ 11. *Pneumocystis*

_____ 12. *M. tuberculosis*

_____ 13. *Histoplasma*

_____ 14. *Escherichia coli*

_____ 15. *Giardia*

_____ 16. *Salmonella*

_____ 17. *Clostridium*

CIRCLE THE CORRECT WORDS

Circle the correct word from the choices provided to complete these sentences.

18. A complex multicellular mass of microorganisms is called a (biofilm, mycosis).

19. (Endotoxins, Exotoxins) are released during bacterial growth, but (endotoxins, exotoxins) are released when the bacteria die.

20. Bacteria that have a (capsule, nucleus) are difficult to phagocytize.

21. Antigenic variation helps a pathogen to (reproduce much more rapidly, avoid recognition by the host).

22. An individual is (allergic, sensitized) when an adequate amount of antibodies or T cells is available to cause a noticeable reaction on reexposure to the antigen.

23. Immediate hypersensitivity reactions initially involve (antibodies, cells), but delayed hypersensitivity reactions initially involve (antibodies, cells).

24. In antibody-dependent cell-mediated cytotoxicity, (NK cells, neutrophils) kill the target cells.

25. Defective tolerance is a factor in development of (type II hypersensitivity, autoimmunity).

26. Individuals with type O blood are universal (recipients, donors) because their erythrocytes have (no A and B antigens, both A and B antigens).

27. Graft-versus-host disease occurs in graft recipients who are (immunocompetent, immunocompromised).

28. Histamine released from mast cells causes signs and symptoms of inflammation by binding to (H1, H2) receptors.

29. Although type II hypersensitivity reactions can affect cells by several different mechanisms, they all involve antigens that are expressed in (many different, only specific) tissues.

DESCRIBE THE DIFFERENCES

Describe the difference between each pair of terms.

30. What is the difference between epidemic and pandemic?

31. What is the difference between pathogenicity and immunogenicity?

32. What is the difference between primary and secondary immune deficiency?

ORDER THE STEPS

Sequence the events that occur when HIV infects a host cell.

33. Write the letters here in the correct order of the steps: _____
    A. HIV envelope fuses with host cell membrane, and viral contents enter host cell.
    B. HIV virion in body fluids encounters a susceptible host cell.
    C. New virion is assembled, buds from host cell, matures, and becomes infectious.
    D. Viral enzyme integrase inserts proviral DNA into host cell DNA.
    E. Proviral DNA is transcribed.
    F. Viral enzyme reverse transcriptase converts viral RNA into proviral DNA.
    G. Viral envelope gp120 binds host cell CD4 and a chemokine co-receptor.
    H. mRNA for viral proteins is translated.

Sequence the events that occur during development of a type I hypersensitivity response.

34. Write the letters here in the correct order of the steps: _____
    A. B lymphocytes produce IgE against the allergen.
    B. IgE attaches to mast cells.
    C. Individual has initial exposure to the allergen.
    D. Mast cells degranulate.
    E. IgE circulates in blood.
    F. IgE on mast cells binds allergen.
    G. Individual has additional allergen exposure.
    H. Individual has clinical signs and symptoms of allergy.
    I. Individual has genetic predisposition to allergy.

COMPLETE THE SENTENCES

Write one word in each blank to complete these sentences.

35. Bacteria that grow in complex multicellular masses called _____ have some protection from host immune responses and antibiotics.

36. Bacteria that produce endotoxins are called _____ bacteria because they cause fever.

37. Fungal infections that are localized in healthy individuals can become _____ in immunosuppressed individuals.

38. Bacteria that produce _____ are resistant to many of the penicillins.

39. An infection that transmits from an animal reservoir is called a _____ infection.

40. Gram-_____ bacteria have lipopolysaccharide in the outer membrane that is known as _____.

41. Autoimmunity occurs when the immune system reacts against _____ to such a degree that the person's own tissues are damaged by autoantibodies or autoreactive T cells.

42. Hypersensitivity reactions require _____ against a particular antigen that results in primary and secondary immune responses.

43. Hypogammaglobulinemia is classified as a _____-lymphocyte deficiency.

44. DiGeorge syndrome involves deficient _____-lymphocyte immunity caused by complete or partial lack of the _____.

Chapter **8** **Infection and Defects in Mechanisms of Defense**

45. Antibodies can _____ target cell receptors, as in Graves disease; antibodies also can destroy or _____ receptors, as in myasthenia gravis.

46. Unusual or recurrent severe infections are common indicators of immune _____.

47. The technical term for hives is _____.

EXPLAIN THE PICTURE

Examine the picture of immune complex–mediated hypersensitivity and answer the questions about it.

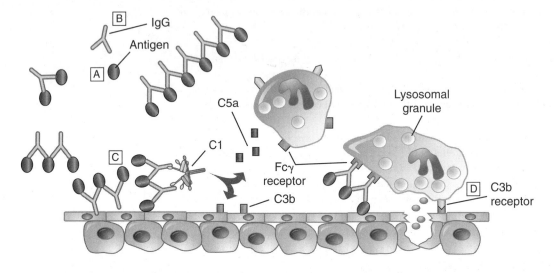

48. Which letter shows the immune complexes? _____

49. What happens to the larger and smaller immune complexes that do not bind to tissue?

50. Why do the neutrophils migrate to this area?

51. What causes the clinical manifestations?

Write your response to each situation in the space provided.

52. Mrs. Desmond says, "If viruses reproduce inside cells, why should I get a flu shot to make antibodies that are outside the cells?"

53. "The doctor said I have an opportunity infection," says Mr. Levine, who has AIDS. "What does that mean?"

54. Billy, age 6, is scheduled for his MMR (measles, mumps, rubella) booster shot. "Why do I have to have this measles shot?" he says. "Mommy said I had this shot when I was a baby."

55. Mrs. Hayes has been HIV positive for 1 year. Her CD4+ cell count is normal. "Wonderful!" she says. "I thought HIV destroyed CD4+ cells. I guess I was wrong."

56. Mr. Lee has AIDS and is hospitalized with dehydration from diarrhea. His nurse wears gloves when cleaning his perineum and emptying his bedpan. "You do not need to wear gloves," he says. "The Internet says that bowel movements do not transmit HIV." How should his nurse respond?

57. Mrs. Hedges took an HIV test after her husband died of AIDS. Her test is positive. "Oh, no!" she exclaims. "Now I have AIDS and am going to die too!"

58. "When immune complexes form, phagocytic cells are supposed to remove them," says a nurse. "Why does immune complex hypersensitivity occur instead?"

59. "What does the *combined* mean in severe combined immunodeficiency disease?" asks Mrs. Quoit, whose son has SCID.

60. "My physician said my cancer drugs gave me a secondary immunodeficiency, so I get sick easily," says Mr. Erie. "I think it is important! Why did she say it is secondary?"

61. "Why not just look at this TB skin test in an hour or so?" says Mr. Rush. "I am going on a business trip tomorrow and cannot come back later this week."

CLINICAL SCENARIOS

Read the clinical scenario and answer the questions to explore your understanding of systemic lupus erythematosus.

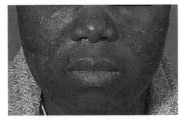

Credit: Forbes CD, Jackson WF: *Color atlas and text of clinical medicine,* ed 3, London, 2003, Mosby.

Ayisha Walker, a 36-year-old woman studying medicine, has aching in her joints (arthralgia) and a new rash on her face. She states that the rash gets worse when she goes out into the sun. She also feels fatigued and gets a sharp pain in her chest when she breathes deeply. She has had "flare-ups" of these symptoms from time to time in the past, but this is the worst episode ever.

PHYSICAL EXAMINATION

- Vital signs normal

- Facial rash over her cheeks and the bridge of her nose

- Discoid scaling red rash on extremities, especially the extensor surfaces of the arms

- Finger and ankle joints with pain and stiffness on passive and active movement

- Chest examination with pleural friction rub heard on deep inspiration

- Cardiac, abdominal, and neurologic examinations normal

- Serum electrolytes normal

- Hematocrit and hemoglobin low; platelet count slightly low; white blood count normal

- Blood urea nitrogen (BUN) and creatinine elevated; protein present in the urine

- Chest radiograph shows a small collection of pleural fluid

- Anti-DNA antibodies positive; antinuclear antibody (ANA) positive

Ms. Walker's diagnosis is systemic lupus erythematosus (SLE).

62. What is the common descriptive term for Ms. Walker's facial rash?

63. Why should Ms. Walker be taught to avoid sunlight?

64. Which of Ms. Walker's laboratory results indicate renal dysfunction? Is renal dysfunction associated with SLE, or is it more likely that she also has a renal disease unrelated to SLE?

65. What other aspects of her history, physical examination, and laboratory results are manifestations of SLE?

66. What does *ANA* mean? Why is it important in SLE?

67. How can SLE cause such widespread tissue damage? What is the pathophysiology?

68. What is a type III hypersensitivity reaction?

9 Stress and Disease

MATCH THE DEFINITIONS

Match each word on the right with its definition on the left.

_____ 1. Chronic overactivation of adaptive regulatory physiologic systems that increases susceptibility to disease

A. Homeostasis

_____ 2. The process of managing stressful challenges that tax the individual's resources

B. Allostasis

_____ 3. Physiologic regulation around a changed or changing set point

C. Allostatic overload

_____ 4. Physiologic regulation around an unchanging set point

D. Coping

IDENTIFY THE EFFECTS OF SYMPATHETIC NERVOUS SYSTEM ACTIVATION

Write increased *or* decreased *beside each item to indicate whether activation of the sympathetic nervous system increases or decreases it from the normal value.*

_____ 5. Heart rate and contractility

_____ 6. Blood pressure

_____ 7. Blood glucose

_____ 8. Skin blood flow

_____ 9. Peristalsis in gastrointestinal tract

_____ 10. Sphincter tone in gastrointestinal tract

_____ 11. Diameter of bronchioles

CIRCLE THE CORRECT WORDS

Circle the correct word from the choices provided to complete these sentences.

12. The general adaptation syndrome is a (specific, nonspecific) response to noxious physiologic stimuli, as described by (Hans Selye, Walter Cannon).

13. Research demonstrates that immune modulation by psychosocial stressors or interventions (leads directly to, does not influence) health outcomes.

14. Epinephrine (increases, decreases) blood levels of free fatty acids.

15. The cortisol effect on protein metabolism is (anabolic, catabolic) in the liver and (anabolic, catabolic) in muscle and other tissues.

16. Cortisol (decreases, increases) blood glucose and (decreases, increases) secretion of gastric acid.

17. Adverse life events that have a large negative impact on immunity are those that are perceived as (predictable, uncontrollable).

45

CATEGORIZE THE CLINICAL SITUATIONS

Write the type of stress response beside each situation. Choices: reactive, anticipatory.

_____ 18. Man develops pounding heart, dry mouth, and shaking hands when his boss tells him he is fired from his job.

_____ 19. Student develops pounding heart, dry mouth, and shaking hands halfway through an examination.

_____ 20. Student develops pounding heart, dry mouth, and shaking hands the night before an examination, while studying.

_____ 21. Woman develops pounding heart, dry mouth, and shaking hands after finding a rat in her apartment building garbage area.

_____ 22. Boy develops pounding heart, dry mouth, and shaking hands when his brother tells him that a monster is under his bed.

_____ 23. Woman develops pounding heart, dry mouth, and shaking hands in the car on the way to her chemotherapy appointment.

EXPLAIN THE PICTURE

Examine the picture and answer the questions about it.

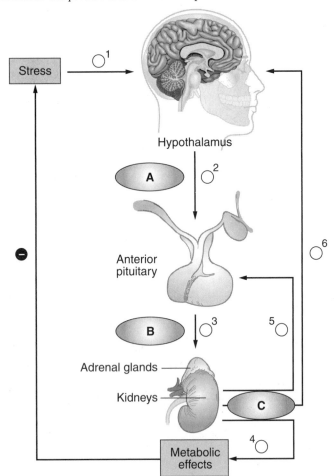

24. Write the names of the hormones represented by the letters.

    A. _____

    B. _____

    C. _____

25. In the circles labeled 1 through 6, write either + (plus) or – (minus) to indicate whether the process is activating or inhibitory.

26. What two-word physiology term is used for the inhibitory effects noted in this picture?

    _____

27. Which numbered circle shows the potentially deleterious actions on the body that occur with chronic stress? _____

IDENTIFY THE EFFECTS OF SLEEP DEPRIVATION

Write increases *or* decreases *by each item to indicate whether sleep deprivation increases or decreases it from the normal value.*

_____ 28. Cortisol levels in blood before the usual bedtime

_____ 29. Blood pressure

_____ 30. Blood glucose

_____ 31. Proinflammatory cytokines

_____ 32. Activity of parasympathetic neurons

COMPLETE THE SENTENCES

Write one word in each blank to complete these sentences.

33. When a physiologic or psychological demand exceeds an individual's coping abilities, the individual experiences _____.

34. The study of how consciousness, the nervous system, and the immune system interact is called _____.

35. The hypothalamic hormone called _____-releasing hormone activates both the _____ axis and the _____ nervous system.

36. The adrenal _____ is an extension of the sympathetic nervous system.

37. Norepinephrine in the brain promotes arousal, _____ vigilance, and _____ anxiety.

38. The hormone _____ that has increased release during the response to stressors is believed to promote social attachment.

39. Poor wound healing occurs in people who have elevated _____ levels.

40. With increasing age, changes in stress-related physiology can _____ an individual's adaptive reserve.

TEACH PEOPLE ABOUT PATHOPHYSIOLOGY

Write your response to each situation in the space provided.

41. A nurse asks, "When I bring the oximeter into the room, why do some of my patients get a sympathetic response with tachycardia and others do not?"

42. "How is it possible for stress to affect immunity?" asks a nurse. "Immune cells are not connected to sympathetic nerves; they are moving around in the body."

43. Farley, age 11, receives outpatient chemotherapy. "Why does my heart pound when I have to come to the hospital for chemo?" he says. "It is scary enough without my heart pounding so fast!"

44. "When I get stressed, my allergies always get worse," says Mr. Williams. "I know my allergies involve antibodies, but I would like to know how being stressed makes my allergies worse."

10 Biology of Cancer

NAME THE NEOPLASMS

Match the description on the right with the neoplasm name on the left.

_____ 1. Lipoma	A. Malignant tumor arising from connective tissue
_____ 2. Sarcoma	B. Malignant tumor of glandular epithelium
_____ 3. Carcinoma	C. Malignant tumor of fat cells
_____ 4. Osteogenic sarcoma	D. Malignant tumor of skeletal muscle
_____ 5. Rhabdomyoma	E. Benign tumor of fat cells
_____ 6. Liposarcoma	F. Benign tumor of smooth muscle
_____ 7. Adenocarcinoma	G. Malignant bone tumor
_____ 8. Leiomyoma	H. Benign tumor of skeletal muscle
_____ 9. Rhabdomyosarcoma	I. Malignant tumor arising from epithelial tissue

COMPLETE THE CHART

Fill in the blank spaces within the chart to compare and contrast the characteristics of benign and malignant tumors.

Characteristic	Benign Tumors	Malignant Tumors
Appearance of the Cells	Well differentiated	
Usual Rate of Growth	Slow	
Mitotic Index		
Presence of Capsule		
Vascularization	Slight	
Mode of Growth	Expansile	
Ability to Metastasize		

CIRCLE THE CORRECT WORDS

Circle the correct word from the choices provided to complete these sentences.

10. Mutations in (oncogenes, proto-oncogenes) that convert them to (oncogenes, proto-oncogenes) drive development of cancer by causing uncontrolled cell growth.

11. If the cancer stem cells in a tumor survive cytotoxic chemotherapy, the tumor is likely to (self-destruct, regrow).

12. Progression from a benign polyp to a malignant tumor requires (multiple, one or two) mutations.

13. The normal (oncogene, proto-oncogene) *ras* becomes the (oncogene, proto-oncogene) *ras* when a mutation makes the RAS protein active all the time.

14. Malignant tumors in the colon most commonly metastasize to the (lungs, liver).

15. Malignant tumors are (heterogeneous, homogeneous) in their cellular composition.

16. In the presence of oxygen, normal cells metabolize glucose by (glycolysis, oxidative phosphorylation), but cancer cells often metabolize it by (glycolysis, oxidative phosphorylation).

17. For a cell to become cancerous, numerous mutations must occur in its (genes, enzymes) (simultaneously, over time).

18. (Acute, Chronic) inflammation predisposes to development of cancer.

MATCH THE DEFINITIONS

Match the word on the right with its definition on the left.

_____ 19. Having variable size and shape

_____ 20. The process by which a cell develops a specialized organization and function

_____ 21. Having no cellular differentiation

_____ 22. The process by which a normal cell becomes a cancer cell

_____ 23. A new growth

_____ 24. Abnormal growth resulting from uncontrolled proliferation

A. Anaplastic

B. Neoplasm

C. Transformation

D. Differentiation

E. Pleomorphic

F. Tumor

CATEGORIZE THE CHANGES

Write the potential effect of the genetic change beside its description. Choices: procancer effect, anticancer effect.

_____ 25. Point mutation inactivates one tumor suppressor gene allele, epigenetic change silences the other.

_____ 26. Chromosome translocation creates Philadelphia chromosome.

_____ 27. Point mutation inactivates proto-oncogene.

_____ 28. Decreased expression of specific noncoding RNAs causes increased expression of oncogenes.

_____ 29. Gene amplification creates multiple copies of gene for epidermal growth factor receptor.

_____ 30. DNA methylation occurs in the promoter regions of both copies of a tumor suppressor gene.

_____ 31. Epigenetic modification silences an oncogene.

_____ 32. Mutation disrupts caretaker gene.

_____ 33. Chromosome instability causes loss of both copies of tumor suppressor genes.

ORDER THE STEPS

Sequence the events that occur when a carcinoma successfully metastasizes through the blood.

34. Write the letters here in the correct order of the steps: _____
    A. Cancer cells attach to vascular endothelium, attracted by tissue-specific characteristics and survival signals of a premetastatic niche.
    B. Tumor microenvironment drives cell dedifferentiation by epithelial-to-mesenchymal transition, with mutations that enable anchorage independence, increased motility, and secretion of proteases.
    C. Cancer cells circulate, evading the immune system by associating with platelets or other mechanisms.
    D. Cancer cells leave the blood vessel, facilitated by their motility characteristics and vascular remodeling.
    E. Cancer cells secrete chemical signals that co-opt local and circulating cells, creating a new microenvironment where they proliferate.
    F. Cancer cells move into a blood vessel, facilitated by leaky blood vessels created through angiogenesis.

EXPLAIN THE PICTURE

Examine the picture and answer the questions about it.

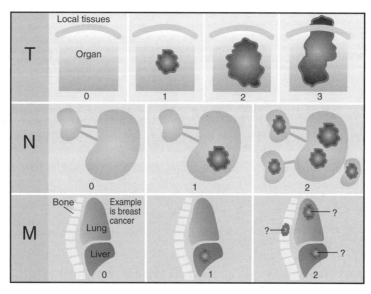

This picture shows the TNM system for breast cancer.

35. What do these letters represent?

    T = _____; N = _____; M = _____

36. Does assigning the TNM numbers grade or stage the cancer? _____

37. Write the TNM numbers for a woman with breast cancer that has metastasized to her lungs, has invaded her chest wall, and has involved several fixed lymph nodes. _____

DESCRIBE THE DIFFERENCES

Describe the difference between each pair of terms.

38. What is the difference between a proto-oncogene and an oncogene?

39. What is the difference between a proto-oncogene and a tumor suppressor gene?

40. What is the difference between a driver mutation and a passenger mutation?

COMPLETE THE SENTENCES

Write one word in each blank to complete these sentences.

41. Stem cells and cancer cells are able to divide indefinitely because they make the enzyme _____.

42. Tumors stimulate formation of new blood vessels by secreting _____ factors.

43. Abnormal premalignant growths in epithelial tissues that have not crossed the basement membrane are called carcinoma _____.

44. Cancer-predisposing genetic events that occur in _____ cells are not inherited, but those that occur in _____ cells are inherited.

45. A cancer cell that secretes growth factors that stimulate its own growth engages in _____ stimulation.

46. Characteristics of cancer cells that enable them to survive and proliferate include loss of contact _____, resistance to apoptosis, and anchorage _____.

47. Survival of malignant tumors is facilitated by tumor-associated _____ that secrete cytokines and other factors that assist cancer cell survival and proliferation.

48. The immune system is important in protecting against cancers caused by specific _____ infections.

TEACH PEOPLE ABOUT PATHOPHYSIOLOGY

Write your response to each situation in the space provided.

49. "My uncle has liver cancer and so does my mom," says Sandi Mauntz. "But the doctor said his cancer is primary and hers is metastatic. What does that mean?"

50. Mr. Winslow has small cell carcinoma of the lung, with persistent hyponatremia. "The doctor told me that cancer cells are making a hormone and said 'paraneoplastic syndrome,' but then her beeper rang and she had to leave in a hurry," says Mrs. Winslow. "Please finish the explanation. What hormone? What does *paraneoplastic syndrome* mean?"

51. "What is the Warburg effect?" says Nurse Davidson, who is reading a journal article about new cancer treatments. "What does that mean?"

52. "Now please explain the reverse Warburg effect," says Nurse Davidson. "Does that mean the cancer cells make glucose instead of burning it for energy?"

CLINICAL SCENARIOS

Read the clinical scenarios and answer the questions to explore your understanding of cancer.

Ms. Lavenia Smith, age 67, went to see her family physician because of dyspnea and a chronic cough. When asked, Ms. Smith stated that she has smoked cigarettes since she was a teenager. Pulmonary function tests show a definite blockage in her airflow; a chest radiograph shows a lesion; and bronchoscopy washings contain malignant cells. Her diagnosis is bronchogenic lung cancer. Histologically, it is a squamous cell carcinoma.

53. Why did Ms. Smith have a blockage in her airflow?

54. Did Ms. Smith's lung cancer metastasize from cancer in another location in her body, or did it arise in her lungs? What information provides this answer?

55. Why did Ms. Smith develop dyspnea?

56. The lining of the bronchi normally is pseudostratified columnar epithelium, not squamous cells. Why did Ms. Smith's cancer develop from squamous cells?

Ms. Smith is scheduled for surgery, followed by radiation therapy and chemotherapy. Surgery will remove the bulk of the tumor, and the radiotherapy is expected to shrink remaining lung tumor cells. The chemotherapy is aimed at metastatic liver tumors that were discovered. Ms. Smith has stopped smoking.

57. Why did Ms. Smith's physician order a liver scan when he discovered that Ms. Smith had bronchogenic carcinoma?

58. Why had Ms. Smith's cancer metastasized before she had enough signs and symptoms to seek out her physician?

Mrs. Gillespie died from stage IV colon cancer. Her son Tom, age 52, was diagnosed with stage I colon cancer that was treated successfully with surgery and chemotherapy. Mr. Gillespie has a lot of questions as he reflects on his experiences.

59. "My mother had stage IV cancer and she died; I had stage I cancer and I survived," says Mr. Gillespie. "Obviously stage IV is worse, but how do the doctors determine what stage a cancer is?"

60. "I remember the oncologist telling my sister and me that our mother's cancer had spread to her liver. What was that fancy 'meta-' word that he used?" says Mr. Gillespie.

61. Mr. Gillespie asks, "Does everybody who gets liver cancer have cancer someplace else first?"

62. "I am grateful that I survived chemotherapy," says Mr. Gillespie. "I knew I would lose my hair, but I was surprised when I got those painful sores in my mouth. How did the chemo cause the sores?"

63. Mr. Gillespie says, "I got so tired during the chemo. My doctor said I was anemic. Did the chemo kill off my red blood cells too?"

64. "My mother had a lot of pain, but the nurses managed the pain medications very well," says Mr. Gillespie. "What surprised me is that I did not have any pain, except from the surgery and those mouth sores. Why didn't I have cancer pain?"

11 Cancer Epidemiology

MATCH THE DEFINITIONS

Match each word on the right with its definition on the left.

_____ 1. Smoke exhaled by a smoker

_____ 2. Smoke from the burning end of a cigarette, cigar, or pipe

_____ 3. Smoke from the burning end of a cigarette, cigar, or pipe plus the smoke exhaled by the smoker

A. Sidestream smoke

B. Environmental tobacco smoke

C. Mainstream smoke

CIRCLE THE CORRECT WORDS

Circle the correct word from the choices provided to complete these sentences.

4. Epigenetic changes that (silence, activate) tumor suppressor genes by DNA (breakage, methylation) facilitate cancer initiation and progression.

5. Infiltration of (red blood, immune) cells supports the progression of a malignant tumor.

6. The leading cause of preventable death in the United States is (cigarette smoking, alcohol abuse).

7. Studies suggest that malnutrition can (increase, decrease) repair of DNA.

8. Chemicals that are not synthesized in the body but may be found in foods are called (xenobiotics, nutrigenomics).

9. Insulin-like growth factor 1 (IGF-1) regulates cell division and has (apoptotic, anti-apoptotic) effects that (increase, decrease) the risk for several types of cancers.

10. Obesity (decreases, increases) the risk for numerous types of cancers.

CATEGORIZE THE DIETARY FACTORS

Write the type of cellular effect beside each dietary factor. Choices: procancer, anticancer.

_____ 11. Lycopene from tomatoes

_____ 12. Polyphenols from tea

_____ 13. *N*-nitroso compounds from nitrites

_____ 14. Organosulfur compounds from garlic

_____ 15. Aflatoxin from moldy peanuts

COMPLETE THE SENTENCES

Write one word in each blank to complete these sentences.

16. Cancer-causing substances are called _____.

17. The term _____ means the study of the interactions between nutrition and an individual's genetic makeup.

18. The degree to which development of a fetus depends on its environment is called developmental _____.

19. Regular exercise _____ the risk for several types of cancers.

20. Adipose tissue releases _____ that influence inflammation and insulin resistance.

21. _____ radiation from sunlight causes _____ cell and squamous cell carcinomas and increases

    the risk for malignant _____.

22. _____ radiation from x-rays and computed tomography scans can initiate premalignant cell changes and promote preexisting ones.

23. _____ increases the risk for malignant mesothelioma and lung cancer; _____ released from

    rocks increases the risk for lung cancer; and inorganic arsenic ingested in _____ increases the risk for bladder and other cancers.

24. Cancer that forms in the skin pigment cells is called malignant _____.

MATCH THE MICROORGANISMS

Match the microorganisms on the right with their associated types of cancers on the left.

_____ 25. Gastric cancer   A. Hepatitis B and C viruses

_____ 26. Cervical cancer   B. *Helicobacter pylori*

_____ 27. Liver cancer   C. Human herpesvirus type 8

_____ 28. Kaposi sarcoma   D. Human papillomavirus types 16 and 18

TEACH PEOPLE ABOUT PATHOPHYSIOLOGY

Write your response to each situation in the space provided.

29. "My doctor said that I should avoid processed foods containing nitrites," says Mrs. Golt, who has a family history of colon cancer. "I know that means hot dogs, but are there others? And what do nitrites have to do with colon cancer anyway?"

30. "I hear that drinking too much alcohol increases the risk for cancer," says Mr. Taylor. "I do not drink hard liquor like vodka or gin. I drink beer, so I am not at risk. Right?"

31. "I heard the radiologist talking about bystander effects," says Mr. Merino, whose cancer is being treated with radiation therapy. "Was someone standing too close to the machine when it was turned on? Or is the machine leaking radiation?"

32. "Help me understand this research about environmental carcinogens," says another nurse. "It talks about transgenerational effects and multigenerational effects. What is the difference?"

12 Cancer in Children and Adolescents

MATCH THE DEFINITIONS

Match each word on the right with its definition on the left.

_____ 1. Leukemia

A. Tumor that originates during fetal life and involves immature cells

_____ 2. Embryonic tumor

B. Malignant eye tumor associated with specific genetic mutations

_____ 3. Wilms tumor

C. Malignant renal tumor associated with congenital abnormalities

_____ 4. Retinoblastoma

D. Malignancy of blood-forming cells

CIRCLE THE CORRECT WORDS

Circle the correct word from the choices provided to complete these sentences.

5. The types of cancers that occur in children and adolescents are (similar to, different from) the types of cancers that occur in adults.

6. Tumors that originate during fetal development and contain immature cells are called (stromal, embryonic) tumors.

7. In general, childhood cancers grow (slowly, rapidly).

8. Mortality rates for childhood cancers have (increased, decreased) significantly in the past 50 years.

9. The letters (oma, blast) in the name of a tumor indicates that it is an embryonic tumor.

CATEGORIZE THE CANCERS

Write the age group with highest incidence beside each type of cancer. Choices: children/adolescents, adults.

_____ 10. Prostate cancer

_____ 11. Brain tumors

_____ 12. Neuroblastoma

_____ 13. Lung cancer

_____ 14. Wilms tumor

_____ 15. Leukemia

MATCH THE RISKS

Match the type of cancer on the right with its potential risk on the left.

_____ 16. Adolescent uses testosterone and related anabolic steroids to increase muscle mass

_____ 17. Child has Fanconi anemia.

_____ 18. Adolescent's mother received DES during pregnancy.

_____ 19. Child has *MYCN* oncogene.

A. Acute myelogenous leukemia

B. Vaginal adenocarcinoma

C. Neuroblastoma

D. Hepatocellular carcinoma

COMPLETE THE SENTENCES

Write one word in each blank to complete these sentences.

20. The most common type of cancer in children is _____.

21. Cryptorchidism (undescended testicles) is a risk factor for _____ cancer.

22. Children who have Down syndrome have increased risk for developing acute _____.

23. Children who have AIDS have increased risk for developing _____ sarcoma and non-Hodgkin _____.

24. Retinoblastoma and Wilms tumor are associated with disabled _____ genes.

TEACH PEOPLE ABOUT PATHOPHYSIOLOGY

Write your response to each situation in the space provided.

25. Mr. Johnson's 2-year-old daughter has been diagnosed with neuroblastoma. He says, "I know that many adult cancers are linked with chemicals in the environment. Why can't the doctors tell us what chemicals are linked with her kind of cancer so that we can have our house tested for them?"

26. "The doctor said Calvin's cancer came from the mesodermal germ layer," says Mrs. Klughart, whose young son has cancer. "What does that mean? Was there an infection?"

27. Mr. Talison's son has just received a cancer diagnosis. "Oh, no! My son has cancer! Now he is going to die!" he says.

28. Another nurse is reading a research study that links exposure to pesticides to development of leukemia. "A big percentage of the children who were exposed to pesticides did develop leukemia, but some of them did not," she says. "So how can I interpret this study?"

29. An oncology nurse who works with adults says, "I see carcinomas commonly in my adult population but I just learned that children rarely develop carcinomas. Why not?"

13 Structure and Function of the Neurologic System

MATCH THE DEFINITIONS

Match each word on the right with its definition on the left.

_____	1. A bundle of axons	A. Axon
_____	2. Protective membranes surrounding brain and spinal cord	B. Corpus callosum
_____	3. Brain system that includes the amygdala, hippocampus, and thalamus	C. Myelin
_____	4. Composed of the midbrain, pons, and medulla oblongata	D. Tract
_____	5. Insulating lipid material that surrounds axons	E. Vagus
_____	6. Neuron extension that carries impulses away from the cell body	F. Meninges
_____	7. Neuron extension that carries impulses toward the cell body	G. Optic
_____	8. The structure that connects the cerebral hemispheres	H. Brainstem
_____	9. Cranial nerve II	I. Dendrite
_____	10. Cranial nerve X	J. Limbic

EXPLAIN THE PICTURES

Examine the pictures and answer the questions about them.

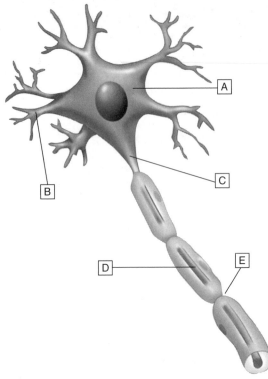

Credit: From Patton KT, Thibodeau GA: *Anatomy & physiology,* ed 8, St Louis, 2013, Mosby.

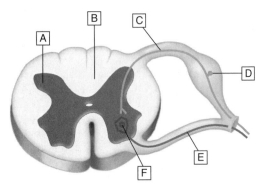

Credit: From Patton KT, Thibodeau GA: *Anatomy & physiology,* ed 8, St Louis, 2013, Mosby.

11. Which letter in the picture indicates an axon?

_____

12. Which letter in the picture indicates a dendrite?

_____

13. Which letter indicates the location where an action potential begins? _____

14. Name the location where an action potential begins.

_____

15. Draw an arrow on the picture to indicate which way the action potential normally travels.

16. Is this neuron unipolar, bipolar, or multipolar?

_____

17. Name the structure marked E in the picture.

_____

18. What is the benefit of having this type of structure on neurons?

19. Which letter in the picture of the spinal cord indicates the cell body of a sensory neuron? _____

20. Which letter in the picture indicates the cell body of a motor neuron? _____

21. What neural structures are marked C and E?

_____

22. Why is the area marked A darker in color than the area marked B?

CIRCLE THE CORRECT WORDS

Circle the correct word from the choices provided to complete these sentences.

23. Neurons (need, do not need) insulin in order to take in glucose.

24. The principle of synaptic (malleability, plasticity) indicates that the central nervous system is capable of change throughout life.

25. An example of (convergence, divergence) is a primary afferent neuron whose axons synapse with several spinal cord neurons at different levels of the spinal cord.

26. The epidural space is (potential, real) in the skull and (potential, real) in the spinal cord.

27. The basal ganglia are part of the (pyramidal, extrapyramidal) pathways.

28. Cell bodies of spinal lower motor neurons are located in the (white, gray) matter of the spinal cord; their axons synapse with (skeletal, vascular smooth) muscles.

29. The thoracolumbar division of the autonomic nervous system is (sympathetic, parasympathetic), and the craniosacral division is (sympathetic, parasympathetic).

30. The term *adrenergic* refers to (sympathetic, parasympathetic) nerves that are (preganglionic, postganglionic, both preganglionic and postganglionic).

CATEGORIZE THE PHYSIOLOGIC EFFECTS

Write the branch of the autonomic nervous system whose stimulation would cause each effect. Choices: sympathetic, parasympathetic.

_____ 31. Increased diameter of pupils

_____ 32. Dry mouth

_____ 33. Contraction of bladder detrusor muscle

_____ 34. Increased plasma free fatty acids

_____ 35. Bradycardia

_____ 36. Increased salivation

_____ 37. Cool, pale skin

_____ 38. Hyperglycemia

_____ 39. Dilation of bronchioles

_____ 40. Increased blood pressure

_____ 41. Increased peristalsis in intestines

Chapter **13** **Structure and Function of the Neurologic System**

ORDER THE STRUCTURES

Start with the skin and place the structures in their anatomic order moving inward to the cerebral cortex.

42. Write the letters here in the correct order of the structures: _____
    A. Skin
    B. Pia mater
    C. Periosteum externum
    D. Subarachnoid space
    E. Dura mater
    F. Arachnoid mater
    G. Skull
    H. Subdural space
    I. Cerebral cortex
    J. Muscle

MATCH THE FUNCTIONS

Match the functions with the brain areas designated by letters.

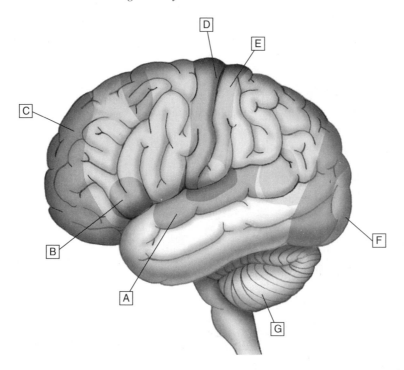

_____ 43. Voluntary motor movement

_____ 44. Vision

_____ 45. Goal-oriented behavior, decision making

_____ 46. Touch and other sensations

_____ 47. Hearing

_____ 48. Motor coordination

_____ 49. Speech

DESCRIBE THE DIFFERENCES

Describe the difference between each pair (or group) of terms.

50. What is the difference between efferent nerves and afferent nerves?

51. What is the difference between the somatic nervous system and the autonomic nervous system?

52. What is the difference between a gyrus, a sulcus, and a fissure in the brain?

53. What is the difference between the anatomic routes that the cranial nerves and the spinal nerves travel to exit the central nervous system on their way to the periphery of the body?

54. What is the difference between an EPSP and an IPSP?

COMPLETE THE SENTENCES

Write one word in each blank to complete these sentences.

55. The peripheral nervous system consists of _____ pairs of spinal nerves and 12 pairs of _____ nerves.

56. The general term for nervous system cells that are not neurons is _____.

57. In the central nervous system, _____ form the myelin sheaths, but in the peripheral nervous system _____ _____ form the myelin sheaths.

58. Groups of cell bodies in the peripheral nervous system are called _____, but groups of cell bodies in the central nervous system are called _____.

59. The _____ plexuses produce cerebrospinal fluid, which returns to the blood at the _____ villi.

60. In a synapse, the space between the two neurons is called the synaptic _____.

61. The _____ body secretes melatonin.

62. Neurons with cell bodies in the substantia nigra use _____ as a neurotransmitter.

63. The technical word for motor nerves crossing contralaterally in the medulla oblongata is _____.

64. When an axon in the peripheral nervous system is severed, a process called _____ degeneration occurs, causing the axon to disappear and the _____ cells to line up in a pathway that facilitates nerve regeneration.

65. Cranial nerves III, IV, and VI are necessary for normal movement of the _____; cranial nerve XII is necessary for normal movement of the _____; cranial nerve _____ is necessary to shrug the shoulders normally against resistance.

TEACH PEOPLE ABOUT PATHOPHYSIOLOGY

Write your response to each situation in the space provided.

66. "When my father had a stroke that affected his left arm and leg, the doctor said the stroke was in the right side of my father's brain," says Mr. Yarrow. "But my cousin lost coordination of the left side of her body after injury to her cerebellum, and the doctor said the injury was on the left side, not the right side. Is one of the doctors wrong?"

67. Mrs. Goldblatt may have trigeminal nerve injury. What tests should be used to assess her trigeminal nerve function?

68. "All these names are so confusing!" says a new nurse. "Rubrospinal tract, spinothalamic tract! How can I remember where they go so I can understand what happens if they are damaged?"

69. Mrs. Kastor's son has a recent head injury and is in the hospital. "Why did they tell me to be sure his neck is straight and his head does not lean to the side?" she asks.

14 Pain, Temperature, Sleep, and Sensory Function

MATCH THE DEFINITIONS

Match each word on the right with its definition on the left.

_____ 1. Inflammation of the cornea	A. Vertigo
_____ 2. Inflammation of the eyelid	B. Chalazion
_____ 3. Cloudy or opaque portion of the lens of the eye	C. Blepharitis
_____ 4. Sensation of spinning around	D. Entropion
_____ 5. Lipogranuloma of oil-secreting gland of the eyelid	E. Keratitis
_____ 6. Eyelid margin turned inward against the eyeball	F. Cataract

CIRCLE THE CORRECT WORDS

Circle the correct word from the choices provided to complete these sentences.

7. A patient who lies on a cold examination table without sufficient padding will lose body heat to the table by (convection, conduction).

8. Non-shivering or chemical thermogenesis occurs when (epinephrine, acetylcholine) acts on (white, brown) fat.

9. Fever (inhibits, increases) many immune defenses against bacteria and viruses.

10. Children develop (lower, higher) fevers than do adults for minor infections; older adults often have (lower, higher) fevers during infection.

11. Heat stroke is characterized by very high body temperature, (presence, absence) of sweat, and (slow, rapid) heart rate.

12. Pain (transmission, transduction) is conversion of chemical or other stimuli into electrical impulses in axons of nociceptors.

13. Normally, REM sleep occurs (before, after) non-REM sleep in a cycle.

CATEGORIZE THE SLEEP DISORDERS

Write the type of sleep disorder beside its name. Choices: dyssomnia, parasomnia. *Then match the examples in the right column with each disorder.*

_____ 14. Insomnia

Example is _____

_____ 15. REM sleep behavior disorder

Example is _____

_____ 16. Somnambulism

Example is _____

_____ 17. Obstructive sleep apnea syndrome

Example is _____

A. Obese man snores and gasps at night and often falls asleep at his computer at work.

B. Woman awakens every night after 2 hours' sleep and has difficulty falling asleep again.

C. Man gets out of bed and acts out his dream while he is dreaming.

D. Child walks around the house while he still is asleep.

EXPLAIN THE PICTURE

Examine the picture and answer the questions about it.

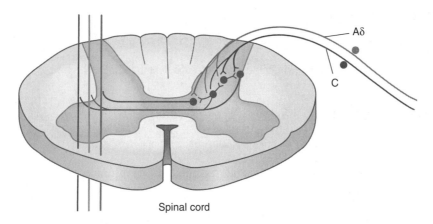

Spinal cord

18. This picture shows pain pathways. Which labeled fibers are unmyelinated? _____

19. What is the clinical significance of the pain pathways crossing to the other side in the spinal cord?

Chapter **14 Pain, Temperature, Sleep, and Sensory Function**

20. What are the names of the tracts in which axons of pain neurons ascend to the brain? _____

21. Which type of pain fiber, A-delta or C, conveys impulses that are interpreted as sharp pain that is highly localized? _____

22. What is the location of the cell bodies of pain neurons that serve as the "gate" for the gate control theory of pain? _____

DESCRIBE THE DIFFERENCES

Describe the difference between each pair of terms.

23. What is the difference between anosmia and ageusia?

24. What is the difference between conductive and sensorineural hearing loss?

25. What is the difference between strabismus and nystagmus?

26. What is the difference between presbycusis and presbyopia?

COMPLETE THE SENTENCES

Write one word in each blank to complete these sentences.

27. The _____ is responsible for thermoregulation and modifies heat production, heat _____, or heat loss mechanisms, based on input from thermoreceptors.

28. The sleep stage in which dreaming occurs is _____.

29. An external hordeolum, commonly called a _____, is infection of the _____ glands of the eyelids.

30. Neonates enter _____ sleep immediately upon falling asleep.

31. Pinkeye is an acute bacterial _____.

32. Papilledema is edema of the _____ nerve where it enters the eyeball and is associated with _____ intracranial pressure.

33. A person who sees double has _____; a person whose eyelid droops has _____.

34. Pain that is felt in an area remote from its point of origin is called _____ pain.

TEACH PEOPLE ABOUT PATHOPHYSIOLOGY

Write your response to each situation in the space provided.

35. "When I started exercising at the gym, the trainer told me not to wipe off my sweat but let it stay on my skin so I would not get heat illness," says Ms. Golan. "Why should I do that? Being sweaty is not ladylike!"

36. "I understand why my patients get fevers from exogenous pyrogens when they have bacterial infections," says another nurse. "But how can a patient who does not have an infection get a mild fever after surgery?"

37. Mr. Smythe is receiving therapeutic hypothermia after a brain injury. His wife says, "I understand why his hand feels so cold, but should I worry because his skin is so pale?"

38. Mr. Nguyen was diagnosed with open-angle glaucoma during a routine eye examination. "I can see fine," he says. "And my eyes do not hurt. Why should I use those glaucoma eyedrops that were prescribed?"

Read each clinical scenario and answer the questions.

Dave Redd, age 25, was hired to do physical labor in a factory near large furnaces that melt metals before processing. After several hours of work, during which his clothes became soaked with sweat, Mr. Redd began to feel weak. He kept working because his supervisor yelled at him when he went to get water and he was afraid he would be fired. Near the end of his shift, Mr. Redd became light-headed and nauseated, and then he fainted. He was taken to the employee health office, which has no laboratory facilities.

Physical Examination

- Blood pressure low, tachycardia, no dysrhythmias, increased respiratory rate, body temperature high

- Skin warm and damp

- Reflexes normal

Mr. Redd's diagnosis is heat exhaustion.

39. Given his diagnosis, should Mr. Redd be positioned lying flat, or should his head and shoulders be elevated? Give a reason for your answer.

40. Why did Mr. Redd develop heat exhaustion?

41. Why did he faint?

42. What caused Mr. Redd's tachycardia?

43. After a short time at the employee health office, Mr. Redd regained consciousness. What type of fluid should he be given to drink?

44. What teaching should the health care provider in the employee health office do to help prevent heat exhaustion in the future?

Mr. Boult, age 61, reports "awful burning pain" in his feet and calves for the past 4 months. He was diagnosed with type 2 diabetes 24 years ago. He manages his diabetes with oral antidiabetic medications.

Physical Examination

- Heart rate, blood pressure, and respiratory rate normal

- Cardiac and abdominal examinations normal

- Skin dry

- Lack of touch sensation in feet and to midpoint of calves bilaterally

Laboratory Results

- Blood glucose and free fatty acids normal

- Serum electrolytes, BUN, and creatinine normal

Mr. Boult's new diagnosis is diabetic neuropathy.

45. What type of pain does diabetic neuropathy cause? _____

46. Why does Mr. Boult not have physiologic manifestations of pain such as tachycardia and elevated blood pressure?

47. What basic physiologic mechanism causes his neuropathic pain? How is that different from nociceptive pain?

15 Alterations in Cognitive Systems, Cerebral Hemodynamics, and Motor Function

MATCH THE DEFINITIONS

Match each word on the right with its definition on the left.

_____ 1. Impaired language production or comprehension that interferes with communication

A. Agnosia

_____ 2. Involuntary rapid contractions of muscle groups in random pattern

B. Athetosis

_____ 3. Impaired recognition of tactile, visual, or auditory patterns

C. Myoclonus

_____ 4. Involuntary rhythmic, oscillating movement of a body part

D. Apraxia

_____ 5. Shocklike, nonpatterned muscle contractions causing limb movement; may occur during sleep

E. Akathisia

_____ 6. Inability to perform purposeful or skilled motor actions

F. Dysphasia

_____ 7. Involuntary slow, twisting, writhing movements

G. Chorea

_____ 8. Motor restlessness, compulsion to move lower extremities

H. Tremor

CIRCLE THE CORRECT WORDS

Circle the correct words from the choices provided to complete these sentences.

9. Cheyne-Stokes respirations involve a cycle of (decreasing, increasing) respiratory rate and depth, then (decreasing, increasing) respiratory rate and depth, and then (dyspnea, apnea) before the cycle begins again.

10. Changes in the pupils are useful to evaluate (cortical, brainstem) function because the areas that control arousal are located (nearby, contralaterally).

11. When autoregulation of intracranial arterioles fails, small increases in blood volume cause intracranial pressure to rise (minimally, greatly).

12. Inflammation from brain injury causes (vasogenic, intracellular) cerebral edema.

13. Hypertonia is caused by damage to (upper, lower) motor neurons when the (upper, lower) motor neurons remain functional.

14. Amyotrophic lateral sclerosis involves degeneration of (upper, lower, both upper and lower) motor neurons.

15. Extrapyramidal motor syndromes involve (abnormal movement, paralysis).

CATEGORIZE THE DYSFUNCTIONS

Write the type of neuromotor dysfunction beside each name. Choices: hyperkinesia, hypokinesia.

_____ 16. Loss of associated movements

_____ 17. Chorea

_____ 18. Akathisia

_____ 19. Bradykinesia

_____ 20. Tremor

_____ 21. Myoclonus

_____ 22. Athetosis

EXPLAIN THE PICTURES

Examine the pictures and answer the questions about them.

A

B

From Rudy EB: *Advanced neurological and neurosurgical nursing,* St Louis, 1984, Mosby.

23. In the posture shown in Figure A, the upper extremities are _____ and the lower extremities are _____ .

24. Figure A shows _____ posture.

25. Interruption of inhibitory messages from what part of the brain is believed to cause this posture? _____

26. In the posture shown in Figure B, the upper extremities are _____ and the lower extremities are

_____ .

27. Figure B shows _____ posture.

28. This posture is believed to occur from severe damage to the cerebrum and the _____ .

ORDER THE LEVELS OF CONSCIOUSNESS

Sequence the progressive changes that occur when a fully alert individual becomes comatose.

29. Write the letters here in the correct order of decreasing consciousness: _____
    A. Light coma
    B. Disorientation
    C. Lethargy
    D. Confusion
    E. Obtundation
    F. Deep coma
    G. Stupor

DESCRIBE THE DIFFERENCES

Describe the difference between each pair of terms.

30. What is the difference between hyperkinesia and hypertonia?

31. What is the difference between arousal and awareness?

32. What is the difference between delirium and dementia?

33. What is the difference between paralysis and paresis?

34. What is the difference between paraplegia and hemiplegia?

COMPLETE THE SENTENCES

Write one word in each blank to complete these sentences.

35. When continuous seizures last more than 5 minutes, the person is said to have _____ _____.

36. Seizure activity often begins in an epileptogenic _____ where the neurons are activated easily.

37. Obstruction of the flow of cerebrospinal fluid causes _____.

38. When intracranial pressure equals mean systolic blood pressure, cerebral blood flow _____.

39. Severely increased intracranial pressure can cause brain tissue to _____ into another cranial compartment.

40. Huntington disease is an autosomal _____ condition characterized by progressive loss of cognitive function, _____ motor movements, and emotional lability.

41. Lower motor neuron damage causes muscle _____, but upper motor neuron damage causes _____.

42. Supratentorial lesions are located above the tentorium _____.

43. Yawning and hiccups are motor responses integrated in the lower _____.

44. A person in a persistent _____ state is unaware of self or environment and has lost all cognitive function but maintains blood pressure and breathing without support.

CLINICAL SCENARIOS

Read each clinical scenario and answer the questions.

Jason Bowen, age 59, has type 2 diabetes that has not been managed well with oral medication. Recently his physician added insulin to his medication regimen. Mr. Bowen accidentally injected too much insulin and had a tonic-clonic seizure, which his wife saw and called an ambulance. After Mr. Bowen has been stabilized in the hospital emergency department, Mrs. Bowen is crying in the hall. "I cannot bear any more!" she says. "First he gets diabetes and now he has epilepsy!"

Physical Examination

- Vital signs normal

- Level of consciousness decreased: confused, disoriented to time and place but not person

- Obese, with abdominal fat distribution

Laboratory Results

- Initial blood glucose in ambulance: 46 mg/dL

- Blood glucose after treatment: 116 mg/dL

Mr. Bowen's admission diagnoses are hypoglycemic seizure and type 2 diabetes.

45. How should a nurse respond to Mrs. Bowen?

46. Did Mr. Bowen have a partial or a generalized seizure? What is the pathophysiologic difference between these two types?

47. What is the "tonic" part of the seizure?

48. What is the "clonic" part of the seizure?

49. Why did Mr. Bowen's confusion and disorientation not resolve immediately when he received intravenous glucose?

50. After he recovered that afternoon, Mr. Bowen said his leg and arm muscles were aching. What most likely caused his muscle aching?

Mrs. Czerny, age 81, was diagnosed with Alzheimer disease when she had difficulty learning the names of her new grandchildren and then got lost several times on the way to her local grocery store. Her family had noticed several years of increasing forgetfulness before her diagnosis but had thought that was part of aging. Over the next 4 years after diagnosis, Mrs. Czerny became more in need of care, because of decreased judgment and self-care ability, and her family hired a full-time caregiver. Eventually, she failed to recognize her family members when they came to visit her, which distressed them greatly. A nurse referred them to a family support group, which they found very helpful.

51. What two classic pathologic changes that contribute to neuronal death are visible in the brain tissue of a person who had Alzheimer disease? Describe each briefly.

52. How soon do clinical manifestations of Alzheimer disease arise after the pathologic changes in the brain begin?

53. Mrs. Czerny's initial symptom was forgetfulness, which is the most common initial manifestation of Alzheimer disease. What portion of her brain was most affected by the pathologic changes at that time?

54. "First she kept forgetting, and now she has poor judgment too," said Mrs. Czerny's son. "I understand that the memory part of her brain is damaged, but now I see more problems. How is this possible?" How should a nurse respond?

Mr. Armstrong, age 73, has advanced Parkinson disease. His disease has progressed until his medications do not control all of the clinical manifestations. He fell this morning and landed on his right side. His wife called an ambulance, which took him to the emergency department. Admission assessment is as follows:

Physical Examination and Subjective Data

- Heart rate, respiratory rate, and blood pressure elevated

- Speaks very softly, with slow response

- Reports right hip pain at a level of 8 on a 0 to 10 scale (10 is worst pain) but has no facial expression of pain

- Bilateral pill-rolling resting tremor of hands, more pronounced on right

- Remainder of examination delayed until return from Radiology

Laboratory Results

- Radiograph: right broken femoral head

- Serum electrolytes normal, blood glucose slightly elevated

Mr. Armstrong's admission diagnoses are right hip fracture, Parkinson disease.

55. What clinical manifestations of Parkinson disease put Mr. Armstrong at risk for falling?

56. Is Parkinson disease a pyramidal or extrapyramidal disorder? What basic pathophysiology causes the motor manifestations of Parkinson disease?

57. Why is Mr. Armstrong speaking so softly?

58. A nurse says, "He says he is in pain, but his face does not show it. Maybe he does not need this pain medication." What is the appropriate response?

16 Disorders of the Central and Peripheral Nervous Systems and the Neuromuscular Junction

MATCH THE DEFINITIONS

Match each word on the right with its definition on the left.

_____ 1. Forward displacement of a vertebra

_____ 2. Degeneration of vertebral structure

_____ 3. Abnormal narrowing of the spinal canal

_____ 4. Disorder of spinal nerve root

A. Radiculopathy

B. Spinal stenosis

C. Spondylolysis

D. Spondylolisthesis

CIRCLE THE CORRECT WORDS

Circle the correct words from the choices provided to complete these sentences.

5. A person who is hit forcefully in the back of the head with a bat can sustain a (coup, contrecoup) injury when the brain hits the front of the skull and a (coup, contrecoup) injury where the bat hit.

6. Subdural hematomas typically involve (arterial, venous) bleeding.

7. (Infection, Hyperactivity) is a significant complication of a compound skull fracture.

8. In diffuse axonal injury, the axons are damaged by (stretching and tearing, penetrating injury).

9. Vertebral injuries tend to occur at the most (rigid, mobile) portions of the vertebral column.

10. Migraine causes (unilateral, bilateral) head pain.

11. Blood in the subarachnoid space after hemorrhage causes (infection, inflammation) and can (impair, potentiate) circulation of cerebrospinal fluid.

12. Hyperextension and hyperflexion vertebral injuries most often occur in the (cervical, lumbar) spine.

13. Most cases of encephalitis are caused by (bacteria, viruses).

14. Brain tumors cause both local and (focal, generalized) effects.

15. Activation of the trigeminal vascular system is an important part of the pathophysiology of (tension, migraine) headaches.

COMPLETE THE CHART

Fill in the blank spaces within the chart to compare and contrast the functions after a spinal cord injury, during the period of spinal shock, and after the return of reflexes.

Function Below the Level of a Complete Spinal Cord Lesion	During the Period of Spinal Shock	After Return of Reflexes
Reflexes		
Motor	_____ paralysis	_____ paralysis
Sensory		
Bladder	Atonic	
Bowels	Atonic	

DRAW YOUR ANSWERS

Read the questions and draw your answers.

16. Draw a saccular aneurysm on this artery.

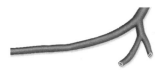

17. Draw a fusiform aneurysm on this artery.

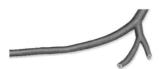

DESCRIBE THE DIFFERENCES

Describe the difference between each pair of terms.

18. What is the difference between a brain contusion and a concussion?

19. What is the difference between mass reflex and autonomic dysreflexia?

20. What is the difference between a myasthenic crisis and a cholinergic crisis in myasthenia gravis?

COMPLETE THE SENTENCES

Write one word in each blank to complete these sentences.

21. Bleeding between the dura mater and the skull causes an _____ hematoma.

22. A classic cerebral concussion is characterized by loss of _____ for less than 6 hours, accompanied by retrograde and anterograde _____ and a confusional state.

23. Release of excitatory neurotransmitters after brain injury causes secondary neural injury known as _____.

24. Neurogenic shock, also called _____ shock, is characterized by bradycardia and _____ blood pressure.

25. Any brain abnormality caused by blood vessel pathophysiology is called _____ disease.

26. The nucleus _____ is the gelatinous inner portion of an intervertebral disk that protrudes if the disk herniates.

27. Clinical manifestations of an ischemic stroke vary, depending on which _____ is obstructed.

28. A person who has a _____ type headache experiences bilateral headache with a sensation of a tight band or pressure around the head.

29. A localized collection of pus in the brain is called a brain _____.

COMPARE THE DEMYELINATING DISORDERS

Compare and contrast multiple sclerosis and Guillain-Barré syndrome by filling in the blank spaces.

Characteristic	Multiple Sclerosis	Guillain-Barré Syndrome
Location of the Demyelinated Axons		
Pathogenesis of the Demyelination		
Signs and Symptoms		
Usual Clinical Course		
Cells That Produce Myelin during Remyelination		

TEACH PEOPLE ABOUT PATHOPHYSIOLOGY

Write your response to each situation in the space provided.

30. Mr. Kanodi is upset. His son Calvin developed an acute subdural hematoma after being hit in the head by a golf ball during a tournament. "Why do they want to make a hole in his skull?" he says. "They could damage his brain!"

31. Mr. Samuels had a thoracic spinal cord injury, and he has completed rehabilitation. His brother says, "I do not understand why he has so many muscle spasms in his legs. My friend had nerve damage in an auto accident and his leg is paralyzed too, but it just lies there flabby-like. Why are my brother's legs so spastic?"

32. Mrs. Kelso, who has multiple sclerosis, says, "Why did it take my doctors 7 years to figure out that my symptoms were caused by multiple sclerosis?"

33. A college campus has an outbreak of meningococcal meningitis. The student health personnel are preparing fliers to post in the dormitories to inform students about signs and symptoms of this infection. What two major signs and symptoms should they list on the fliers, telling students to seek immediate medical assistance if they occur?

34. Mr. Gardner has an astrocytoma that was discovered when he had a seizure. "What does astrocytoma mean?" asks his wife. "Does that mean his brain cells that transmit messages have made a tumor?"

35. Mrs. Torrentia has newly diagnosed myasthenia gravis. "Tell me again why I start seeing double after I have been awake for several hours," she asks.

Read the clinical scenarios and answer the questions.

Mr. Tom Costa, age 71, had a stroke last year that made his right upper and lower extremities quite weak. He has smoked for 55 years and is obese. He was diagnosed with atrial fibrillation, high blood pressure, and type 2 diabetes mellitus while he was hospitalized with his stroke. His father died of a heart attack at age 50; his paternal grandfather had a stroke and died a year later after a second stroke. His mother and both of her parents had type 2 diabetes.

36. What technical term should be used to describe Mr. Costa's weak right upper and lower extremities?

   _____

37. The lesion that caused his motor dysfunction is located on which side of his brain? _____

38. Given his history, is it more likely that Mr. Costa had an ischemic or a hemorrhagic stroke? _____

39. What is a potential relationship between Mr. Costa's atrial fibrillation and his stroke?

40. What is a potential relationship between Mr. Costa's other risk factors and his stroke?

41. Mrs. Costa says, "Tom's grandfather had a stroke and he could not talk any more, but he could walk. Now my husband has a stroke, and he can talk but he cannot walk. I do not understand this! Why?" Explain to Mrs. Costa.

42. "The doctor said to call her if I had a TIA," says Mr. Costa. "Why should I do that? A TIA goes away." Explain to Mr. Costa.

Mr. Goff, who had a complete T4 spinal cord transection 2 years ago, was admitted today for treatment of a pressure ulcer. While a nurse is obtaining his admission history, Mr. Goff says that he just got a pounding headache and is getting very anxious. His upper body has become flushed.

43. What two words describe the likely reason for Mr. Goff's symptoms? _____

44. What findings should be anticipated when a nurse measures Mr. Goff's blood pressure and heart rate?

   _____

45. What pathophysiologic mechanisms account for the changes in blood pressure and heart rate?

46. What makes this situation potentially life threatening?

47. What are common triggers for this situation?

48. Would those triggers cause this situation in a person who has a T10 injury? Why or why not?

17 Alterations of Neurologic Function in Children

MATCH THE DEFINITIONS

Match each word on the right with its definition on the left.

_____ 1. Protrusion of a portion of brain and meninges through a defect in the skull

_____ 2. Small head circumference with decreased brain growth

_____ 3. Birth defect involving failure of closure of the vertebrae

_____ 4. Malformation of the shape of the skull

A. Spina bifida

B. Plagiocephaly

C. Encephalocele

D. Microcephaly

CIRCLE THE CORRECT WORDS

Circle the correct word from the choices provided to complete these sentences.

5. Neural tube defects are associated with maternal (iodine, folate) deficiency.

6. Chiari malformations involve downward displacement of the (cerebellum, motor cortex) and are a type of (defect of neural tube closure, malformation of cortical development).

7. Cerebral palsy is a (progressive, static) encephalopathy.

8. Tethered cord syndrome involving altered (gait and bladder control, speech and cognition) may develop in children born with (myelomeningocele, craniosynostosis) as the child grows.

9. Cerebral palsy is caused by injury or abnormal development in the immature (spinal cord, brain) before, during, or after birth up to (1 year, 5 years) of age.

10. Cerebral palsy always involves (motor, sensory, cognitive) defects and may involve additional problems as well.

11. Febrile seizures in young children are (benign, signs of epilepsy).

CHARACTERIZE THE DISORDERS

Write one letter and one number by each disorder in the left column to indicate the location of damage and the clinical manifestations.

Disorder	Choose the Location of the Damage	Choose the Clinical Manifestations
_____ 12. Dystonic cerebral palsy	A. Neurons throughout the body	1. Increased muscle tone, prolonged primitive reflexes, hyperreflexia, clonus, contractures
_____ 13. Spastic cerebral palsy	B. Basal ganglia, thalamus or cerebellum	2. Purposeful movements are jerky, uncontrolled, abrupt; difficulty with fine motor control
_____ 14. Tay-Sachs disease	C. Corticospinal (pyramidal) pathways	3. Excessive startle response, loss of developmental milestones, seizures, blindness, death

DESCRIBE THE DIFFERENCES

Describe the difference between each pair of terms.

15. What is the difference between a meningocele and a myelomeningocele?

16. What is the difference between pyramidal and extrapyramidal cerebral palsy?

COMPLETE THE SENTENCES

Write one word in each blank to complete these sentences.

17. Children who have congenital arteriovenous malformations are at risk for _____ stroke.

18. Blockage of the cerebral ventricles or aqueduct causes _____ by interfering with the circulation of _____ fluid.

19. Aseptic meningitis may be caused by virus but not by _____.

20. Group _____ *Streptococcus* that causes fatal bacterial meningitis in neonates is transmitted from the mother during _____.

21. Phenylketonuria is caused by mutation of a gene for an _____ that normally converts the _____ acid phenylalanine to _____.

22. Children who have _____ seizures often stare into space, unresponsive, for a few seconds and then resume their activities.

23. A young child who has repeated and worsening headaches should be evaluated for _____ _____ or other cause of increased intracranial pressure.

24. Signs and symptoms of a childhood brain tumor depend on its _____ in the brain and its rate of _____.

TEACH PEOPLE ABOUT PATHOPHYSIOLOGY

Write your response to each situation in the space provided.

25. Tim Jones, age 10, has been diagnosed with epilepsy. His seizures are simple partial seizures. The school nurse is talking with his teacher. "I think he is just faking," says the teacher. "That wasn't a real seizure. If he had a seizure, he would fall down on the ground and twitch all over." How should the nurse respond?

26. Hector, age 2, has pneumococcal meningitis. "My poor sick baby!" says his mother. "Please tell me why he will not bend his neck to drink from his cup of water and why he cried so hard when I tried to straighten his little legs. I am worried that he is paralyzed like my uncle who had a stroke."

27. "My baby used to grasp my finger when I placed it in his palm," says Mrs. Delibes. "That was so cute! But now that he is 6 months old, he does not do that anymore. Is something wrong with him?"

28. Jeannie Quantz, age 4, developed rapidly increasing intracranial pressure during an episode of bacterial meningitis, which blocked her arachnoid villi. Her doctors tell Mrs. Quantz that Jeannie has hydrocephalus and they need to intervene quickly. "Jeannie does not have hydrocephalus!" Mrs. Quantz says to a nurse. "Hydrocephalus is having too much fluid in the brain. My friend who worked in an orphanage overseas showed me pictures of hydrocephalus. Those babies had great big heads from too much fluid inside."

Chapter **17 Alterations of Neurologic Function in Children**

18 Mechanisms of Hormonal Regulation

NAME THE GLANDS AND THEIR HORMONES

Write the name of the gland and the major hormones it secretes beside each number.

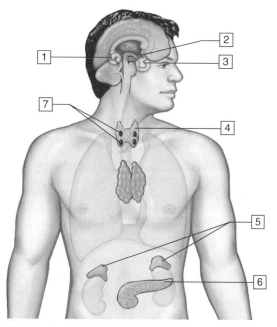

(From Patton KT, Thibodeau GA: *Anatomy & physiology,* ed 9, St Louis, 2016, Mosby.)

1. Gland: _____

   One hormone: _____

2. Gland: _____

   Six hormones: _____

3. Gland: _____

   Seven hormones from anterior: _____

   Two hormones from posterior: _____

4. Gland: _____

   Three hormones: _____

5. Gland: _____

   Three hormones from cortex: _____

   Two hormones from medulla: _____

6. Gland: _____

   Four hormones: _____

7. Gland: _____

   One hormone: _____

MATCH THE DEFINITIONS

Match each word on the right with its definition on the left.

_____ 8. Up-regulation

_____ 9. Permissive effect

_____ 10. Down-regulation

_____ 11. First messenger

_____ 12. Second messenger

A. Chemical signals generated within a cell that mediate the action of a water-soluble hormone or other chemical

B. Water-soluble hormone or other chemical that binds to receptors in plasma membranes

C. Increased numbers or affinity of hormone receptors in response to low hormone concentration

D. Decreased numbers or affinity of hormone receptors in response to high hormone concentration

E. Hormone-induced changes that facilitate the maximal response or functioning of a cell

CATEGORIZE THE HORMONES

Write the type of hormone beside each name. Choices: peptide, steroid, amine.

_____ 13. Cortisol

_____ 14. Insulin

_____ 15. Thyroid hormones

_____ 16. Adrenocorticotropic hormone (ACTH)

_____ 17. Corticotropin-releasing hormone (CRH)

_____ 18. Aldosterone

_____ 19. Glucagon

_____ 20. Growth hormone (GH)

CIRCLE THE CORRECT WORDS

Circle the correct word from the choices provided to complete these sentences.

21. The hypothalamus is connected to the posterior pituitary by (portal blood vessels, a nerve tract) and to the anterior pituitary by (portal blood vessels, a nerve tract).

22. Water-soluble hormones generally have a (short, long) half-life and circulate in (bound, free) forms.

23. Low hormone concentrations usually cause cells to (down-regulate, up-regulate) receptors for that hormone, which (increases, decreases) cellular sensitivity to that hormone.

24. Water-soluble hormones bind with (cell membrane, intracellular) receptors.

25. Hormone receptors are (proteins, steroids, either proteins or steroids).

26. (GH, ACTH) is an example of a somatotropic hormone.

27. (Water, Lipid)-soluble hormones alter gene expression when the hormone-receptor complex binds to the sites on (RNA, DNA) in the (nucleus, ribosomes).

28. Secretion of cortisol increases when (ACTH, CRH) binds to receptors on cells in the adrenal (cortex, medulla).

29. Many of the actions of growth hormone are mediated through the effects of (insulin-like growth factors, incretins, ghrelins), which also are known as (somatotropins, somatomedins, somatostatins).

30. Catecholamines are released from the adrenal (cortex, medulla).

31. The action of catecholamines (increases, decreases) blood glucose concentration as part of the (hypothalamic/pituitary/adrenal axis, fight-or-flight response).

32. The net effect of insulin is to (increase, decrease) blood glucose concentration and (increase, decrease) synthesis of protein and fat.

33. Cortisol acts to (increase, decrease) blood glucose concentration, (stimulate, inhibit) inflammation, and cause (only a few, numerous) other effects.

34. A common mechanism of hormonal regulation is (positive, negative) feedback.

MATCH THE FUNCTIONS

Match the altered function on the right with the hormone on the left.

A Significant Change in Secretion of This Hormone

_____ 35. Antidiuretic hormone (ADH)

_____ 36. Parathyroid hormone (PTH)

_____ 37. Insulin

_____ 38. Gonadotropin-releasing hormone (GnRH)

_____ 39. Aldosterone

Alters the Regulation of This Variable

A. Plasma calcium concentration

B. Blood glucose concentration

C. Body fluid osmolality

D. Extracellular fluid volume and plasma potassium concentration

E. Reproductive cycle regulation

DESCRIBE THE DIFFERENCES

Describe the difference between each pair of terms.

40. What is the difference between a direct effect and a permissive effect of a hormone?

41. What is the difference between autocrine and paracrine action of a hormone?

42. What is the difference between negative and positive feedback?

COMPLETE THE SENTENCES

Write one word in each blank to complete these sentences.

43. Steroid hormones are synthesized from _____.

44. ADH also is called arginine _____.

45. In order for a hormone to act on a cell, the cell must have _____ for that hormone.

46. Hormones that bind to receptors that activate adenylyl cyclase use _____ as a second messenger.

47. Releasing hormones are produced by the _____.

48. An individual who has an iodine-deficient diet will have difficulty making enough _____ hormones.

49. In the islets of Langerhans, alpha cells produce _____, and beta cells produce insulin and _____.

50. Calcitonin is secreted by the _____ gland and helps to regulate plasma _____ concentration.

51. The term *somatopause* indicates the decrease of _____ hormone and insulin-like _____ that occurs with aging.

52. The neurohypophysis is the _____ pituitary, and the adenohypophysis is the _____ pituitary.

Write your response to each situation in the space provided.

53. A clinical research protocol includes drawing blood to measure insulin levels. "Our research subjects do not like blood draws," says a research assistant. "Can we measure urine insulin instead?"

54. "This drug information sheet says that sildenafil prolongs the action of cyclic GMP in blood vessel muscles," says Mr. Lehrner. "I asked my doctor and he said cGMP is a second messenger. What does 'second messenger' mean? Is that an abnormal thing?"

55. Mr. Merryweather has a tumor that damaged his hypothalamus but not his pituitary gland. Among numerous other hormone problems, he is not secreting enough antidiuretic hormone (ADH). "I do not understand this," says a nurse. "ADH comes from the pituitary and does not have a releasing hormone from the hypothalamus. How can his hypothalamic tumor cause his lack of ADH?"

56. "I understand why I need to take this antithyroid drug," says Mr. Henderson, who has newly diagnosed hyperthyroidism. "It stops my thyroid gland from making any more thyroid hormones. But why does it take several weeks to have full effects? Don't we make thyroid hormone every day?"

57. A student is observing in an endocrine clinic. "Why do these laboratory slips have a place to request blood levels of carrier proteins for some hormones like thyroid but not for others like ADH and ACTH?"

58. "Please help me make sense of the renin-angiotensin system," says Mr. Phillipi. "If the kidney blood vessels sense low blood flow, they release renin into the blood, but how does that help fix the low blood flow? I want the details!"

19 Alterations of Hormonal Regulation

MATCH THE DEFINITIONS

Match each word on the right with its definition on the left.

_____ 1. Ectopic hormone   A. Hormone secreted by intestinal endocrine cells

_____ 2. Hirsutism   B. Hormone secreted by nonendocrine tissues

_____ 3. Somogyi effect   C. Nonpitting boggy edema caused by infiltration of mucopolysaccharides and proteins between connective tissue fibers in the dermis

_____ 4. Incretin   D. Excessive growth of facial and body hair

_____ 5. Myxedema   E. Low blood sugar during the night that may lead to morning hypoglycemia

SORT THE DISORDERS

Write the names of the endocrine disorders with their dysfunctioning organs.

Sort these seven disorders: primary hyperthyroidism, secondary hyperthyroidism, SIADH, Cushing disease, diabetes insipidus, primary hypothyroidism, secondary hypothyroidism.

6. Two disorders caused by posterior pituitary dysfunction:

_____

_____

7. Two disorders caused by a problem within the thyroid gland:

_____

_____

8. Three disorders caused by a problem in the anterior pituitary gland:

_____

_____

_____

CIRCLE THE CORRECT WORDS

Circle the correct word from the choices provided to complete these sentences.

9. Syndrome of inappropriate antidiuretic hormone secretion (SIADH) is characterized by (high, low) levels of ADH in the absence of normal control mechanisms.

10. An active anterior pituitary adenoma usually causes (hyposecretion, hypersecretion) of hormones from the adenoma itself and (hyposecretion, hypersecretion) of hormones from the surrounding pituitary cells.

11. Women who have gestational diabetes have (decreased, increased) risk for type 2 diabetes later in life.

12. An individual with type 1 diabetes who has the dawn phenomenon has a (lower, higher) blood glucose in the early morning than in the middle of the night.

13. Metabolic syndrome increases the risk of developing type (1, 2) diabetes.

14. In autoimmune type (1, 2) diabetes, pancreatic beta cells are destroyed by autoreactive (cytotoxic T lymphocytes, natural killer cells).

15. People who have type 1 diabetes have a deficit of insulin and (glucagon, amylin) and a relative excess of (glucagon, amylin).

16. In diabetes, *microvascular disease* refers to damage to (large and medium-sized arteries, capillaries), whereas *macrovascular disease* refers to damage to (large and medium-sized arteries, capillaries).

MATCH THE CLINICAL MANIFESTATIONS

Match the clinical manifestation on the right with the disorder on the left.

_____ 17. SIADH

_____ 18. Hypothyroidism

_____ 19. Pheochromocytoma

_____ 20. Adrenal adenoma causing hypersecretion of androgens in a woman

_____ 21. Diabetic ketoacidosis

_____ 22. Hypoglycemia

_____ 23. Primary hyperaldosteronism

_____ 24. Type 1 diabetes mellitus

_____ 25. Diabetes insipidus

_____ 26. Addison disease

A. Hypertension, tachycardia, palpitations, severe headache, diaphoresis, heat intolerance, weight loss, constipation

B. Polydipsia, nocturia, polyuria, hypernatremia, increased plasma osmolality, large volume of dilute urine

C. Polydipsia, nocturia, polyuria, increased appetite, weight loss, hyperglycemia, glycosuria

D. Weakness, fatigue, hypotension, hyperkalemia, hypoglycemia, elevated ACTH

E. Lethargy, cold intolerance, hoarseness, nonpitting boggy edema around eyes, coarse hair, decreased body temperature

F. Lethargy, hyponatremia, perhaps seizure, decreased plasma osmolality, concentrated urine

G. Tachycardia, diaphoresis, tremor, pallor, confusion, decreased level of consciousness, perhaps seizure

H. Virilization: lack of breast development, hirsutism, increased muscle bulk

I. Polyuria, decreased level of consciousness, Kussmaul breathing, acetone smell to breath, hyperglycemia, decreased blood pH, ketonuria, glycosuria

J. Hypertension, hypokalemia, increased blood pH, increased urine potassium

DESCRIBE THE DIFFERENCES

Describe the difference between each pair of terms.

27. What is the difference between a primary and a secondary endocrine disorder?

28. What is the difference between thyrotoxicosis and thyrotoxic crisis?

29. What is the difference between neurogenic and nephrogenic diabetes insipidus?

30. What is the difference between acromegaly and gigantism?

COMPLETE THE SENTENCES

Write one word in each blank to complete these sentences.

31. Chromaffin cell tumors of the adrenal medulla are called _____.

32. Severe SIADH is associated with _____ serum osmolality and sodium concentration.

33. When necrosis or another problem in the anterior pituitary causes deficiency of all its hormones, the individual has _____.

34. Prolactin-secreting tumors in the _____ pituitary are called _____; in women, they cause _____ (milk production not associated with childbirth).

35. A person who has hypothyroidism can develop a nonpitting boggy edema called _____; that same term, when used with the word *coma,* indicates the _____ level of consciousness associated with severe hypothyroidism.

36. Enlargement of the thyroid gland is called a _____ and is a response to increased stimulation by _____.

37. Type 1 diabetes often is diagnosed when the acute complication _____ _____ occurs.

38. People who have primary hyperparathyroidism are predisposed to form kidney _____.

39. Cushing _____ is caused by hypersecretion of ACTH from the anterior pituitary, but Cushing _____ indicates any condition involving chronic exposure to excessive cortisol.

Examine the picture and answer the questions about it.

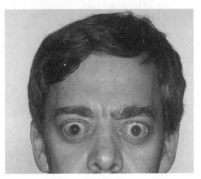

(Belchetz P, Hammond P: *Mosby's color atlas and text of diabetes and endocrinology,* Edinburgh, 2003, Mosby.)

40. What term describes the ophthalmopathy in the photograph? _____

41. With what condition is it associated? _____

42. Why are his eyeballs protruding?

TEACH PEOPLE ABOUT PATHOPHYSIOLOGY

Write your response to each situation in the space provided.

43. A nurse says, "My type 2 diabetes patients do not get diabetic ketoacidosis as often as my type 1 diabetes patients do. Why is that?"

44. Mrs. Soderstrom has newly diagnosed acromegaly. Her husband says, "Last winter I had to buy my wife a larger pair of gloves and larger boots, even though her old ones were in good condition. Our doctor says she has too much growth hormone. Why doesn't too much growth hormone make her tall like a giant?"

45. Mr. James has a pathologic fracture and newly diagnosed hyperparathyroidism. He says, "How can little glands in my neck make my bones weak?"

46. Mrs. King had thyroid surgery yesterday. She says, "Why do the nurses keep blowing up a blood pressure cuff and looking at my hand instead of measuring my blood pressure?"

47. "Dr. Michaels said I have diabetes insipidus," says Mr. Wrey, who has an indwelling urinary catheter. "Diabetes is a sugar problem, but he said my sugar is normal. What is going on?"

48. Mrs. Santos has type 2 diabetes. She says, "Please explain to me why losing weight will help my diabetes."

49. Mr. Parks has newly diagnosed Addison disease. He asks, "Why do I get lightheaded when I stand up?"

CLINICAL SCENARIO

Read the clinical scenario and answer the questions.

Mrs. Mendoza, who has had type 2 diabetes for 17 years, had a below-the-knee amputation of her gangrenous left foot yesterday. Her electronic health record indicates that she has peripheral neuropathy, diabetic retinopathy with loss of visual acuity, gastroparesis, and two previous hospitalizations for hyperosmolar hyperglycemic nonketotic syndrome.

50. What are the two basic components of the pathophysiology of type 2 diabetes?

_____

51. What factors most likely contributed to Mrs. Mendoza's foot needing to be amputated?

52. What is the pathophysiology behind Mrs. Mendoza's diabetic retinopathy?

53. Is diabetic retinopathy a microvascular problem or a macrovascular problem? _____

54. At lunchtime, Mrs. Mendoza says, "I can't eat this lunch! I am still full from breakfast." What complication of diabetes is behind her statement? _____
What two words describe the pathophysiology of this complication? _____ _____ Is this complication a microvascular problem or a macrovascular problem? _____

55. Why should Mrs. Mendoza's urine be checked for microalbuminuria?

56. If Mrs. Mendoza develops hypoglycemia from her medications, what signs and symptoms would be expected?

57. When Mrs. Mendoza developed hyperosmolar hyperglycemic nonketotic syndrome, what signs and symptoms were likely?

58. Mrs. Mendoza's husband says, "The doctor said that my wife has high risk for a heart attack because she has diabetes. How does diabetes contribute to a heart attack?" How should a nurse respond?

59. Why should Mrs. Mendoza's right foot be checked for perfusion as well as skin integrity?

20 Structure and Function of the Hematologic System

MATCH THE DEFINITIONS

Match each word on the right with its definition on the left.

_____ 1. Hemoglobin

_____ 2. Hepcidin

_____ 3. Thrombopoietin

_____ 4. Tissue thromboplastin

_____ 5. Plasmin

_____ 6. Myoglobin

A. Chemical released by damaged cells that activates coagulation

B. Enzyme that dissolves clots

C. Oxygen-binding molecule in muscle cells

D. Oxygen-binding molecule in erythrocytes

E. Hormone growth factor that regulates platelet formation

F. Hormone that regulates iron homeostasis

CLASSIFY THE CELLS

Write the type of cell beside each name. Choices: granulocyte, agranulocyte.

_____ 7. Macrophage

_____ 8. Natural killer cell

_____ 9. Lymphocyte

_____ 10. Neutrophil

_____ 11. Monocyte

_____ 12. Basophil

_____ 13. Eosinophil

CIRCLE THE CORRECT WORDS

Circle the correct word from the choices provided to complete these sentences.

14. Mature erythrocytes (have, do not have) a nucleus; mature neutrophils have a (round, multilobed) nucleus.

15. Neutrophils, basophils, and eosinophils are (immunocytes, granulocytes).

16. The term *hematopoiesis* refers to production of (erythrocytes, blood cells) and occurs primarily in the (bone marrow, spleen) after birth.

17. In the bone marrow, hematopoietic stem cells in the (osteoblastic, vascular) niche are active, but hematopoietic stem cells in the (osteoblastic, vascular) niche are dormant.

18. Each hemoglobin A molecule consists of (two, four) polypeptide chains and (two, four) hemes; in order to bind oxygen, the iron portion of heme must be (ferrous Fe^{2+}, ferric Fe^{3+}).

19. Iron balance is maintained through controlled (absorption, excretion); iron circulates attached to (ferritin, transferrin) and is stored inside cells attached to (ferritin, transferrin).

20. Nitric oxide and prostacyclin (trigger, inhibit) platelet adhesion and aggregation; thromboxane-A_2, epinephrine, thrombin, and collagen (trigger, inhibit) platelet adhesion and aggregation.

MATCH THE FUNCTIONS

Match the cell on the right with its function on the left.

_____ 21. Do active phagocytosis; process and present antigens; participate in wound healing

_____ 22. Process antigens and present them to lymphocytes

_____ 23. Produce antibodies against specific antigens

_____ 24. Kill tumor cells and virus-infected cells

_____ 25. Precursor cells for macrophages

_____ 26. Do phagocytosis early in inflammation; kill bacteria

_____ 27. Defend against parasites

A. Eosinophils

B. Neutrophils

C. Macrophages

D. B lymphocytes (plasma cells)

E. Natural killer cells

F. Dendritic cells

G. Monocytes

NAME THE PROGENITORS

Write the type of progenitor cell beside each mature cell or cell fragment. Choices: lymphoid, myeloid.

_____ 28. Erythrocyte

_____ 29. Natural killer cell

_____ 30. Eosinophil

_____ 31. Monocyte

_____ 32. T cell

_____ 33. Neutrophil

_____ 34. Basophil

_____ 35. Plasma cell (mature B cell)

_____ 36. Platelet

DESCRIBE THE DIFFERENCES

Describe the difference between each pair of terms.

37. What is the difference between a leukocyte and a lymphocyte?

38. What is the difference between plasma and serum?

39. What is the difference between a reticulocyte and an erythrocyte?

40. What is the difference between ferritin and apoferritin?

41. What is the difference between mitosis and endomitosis?

COMPLETE THE SENTENCES

Write one word in each blank to complete these sentences.

42. The most abundant plasma protein is _____; the most abundant leukocytes are the _____.

43. The capacity to be _____ deformed is important for erythrocytes because it enables them to squeeze through the sinusoids of the _____ and through the smallest capillaries.

44. Platelets, also called _____, are cytoplasmic fragments of large cells called _____ that are located in the _____ _____.

45. Erythropoietin stimulates bone marrow to produce more _____; thrombopoietin stimulates bone marrow to produce more _____.

46. Plasmin is an enzyme that degrades _____ polymers; its inactive precursor is _____, which is produced by the _____.

47. Lymphocytes tend to have decreased function in _____ adults.

EXPLAIN THE PICTURE

Examine the picture and answer the questions about it.

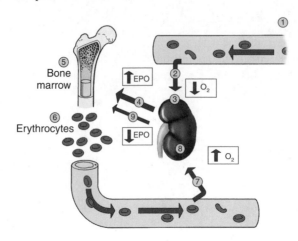

48. What does the acronym EPO mean? _____

49. In the picture, EPO is released by the _____ and acts on the _____ _____.

50. What does EPO stimulate bone marrow to do? _____

51. What causes increased release of EPO? _____

52. Where does negative feedback occur in the picture?

_____

CATEGORIZE THE SUBSTANCES

Write the function of each substance with regard to blood clotting. Choices: promotes clotting, antithrombotic.

_____ 53. Plasminogen activators

_____ 54. Tissue thromboplastin

_____ 55. Thrombomodulin, protein C, and protein S

_____ 56. Tissue factor pathway inhibitor

_____ 57. Exposure of blood to collagen

_____ 58. Thrombin

_____ 59. Prostacyclin

_____ 60. Antithrombin III

_____ 61. Nitric oxide

Write your response to each situation in the space provided.

62. "I had a blood transfusion a few years ago," said Mrs. Wilder. "Every once in a while I worry about that stranger's red cells moving around my body."

63. Mrs. Abbott received an erythropoietin injection to treat her severe anemia. "My physician said my reticulocyte count is increased, which is good," she says. "But aren't reticulocytes immature red blood cells? Why is that good?"

64. "My nurse practitioner told me I need more iron in my diet to help make red blood cells," says Mrs. Jeterman. "What does iron have to do with red blood cells?"

65. "I am reading a mystery story in which the important clue was high bilirubin in a man's blood when a poison caused a lot of his red blood cells to die," says Mrs. Verde. "What do red blood cells have to do with bilirubin?"

66. A nurse says, "I hear that platelets release various chemicals, including some proteins like clotting and growth factors, when they are activated. But protein synthesis takes time, and platelet activation occurs very fast. Please explain this!"

67. Mr. Patel has signs of deep venous thrombosis, and a blood sample was drawn to measure D-dimer. He says, "What is D-dimer? How will measuring it help to decide whether or not I have a blood clot in my leg?"

68. Mr. Howells was injured in a knife fight. His partner says, "I know that scabs eventually fall off. What happens to clots in blood vessels inside the body? Do they fall off into the blood when the blood vessel heals? Wouldn't that cause a problem?"

Alterations of Hematologic Function

MATCH THE DEFINITIONS

Match each word on the right with its definition on the left.

_____ 1. Increased blood level of immature erythrocytes

_____ 2. Increased number or volume of circulating erythrocytes

_____ 3. Decreased number or volume of circulating erythrocytes

_____ 4. Premature death of damaged erythrocytes

_____ 5. Having erythrocytes of different shapes

_____ 6. Having erythrocytes of different sizes

_____ 7. Lower than normal blood counts of white blood cells, red blood cells, and platelets

_____ 8. Enlarged lymph nodes

_____ 9. Lower than normal neutrophil count in the blood

_____ 10. Complete absence of neutrophils, eosinophils, and basophils in the blood

_____ 11. Higher than normal white blood cell count

_____ 12. Lower than normal white blood cell count

_____ 13. Higher than normal blood counts of neutrophils, eosinophils, and basophils

_____ 14. Lower than normal blood counts of neutrophils, eosinophils, and basophils

A. Anemia

B. Anisocytosis

C. Poikilocytosis

D. Pancytopenia

E. Reticulocytosis

F. Eryptosis

G. Polycythemia

H. Granulocytopenia

I. Leukopenia

J. Lymphadenopathy

K. Granulocytosis

L. Agranulocytosis

M. Leukocytosis

N. Neutropenia

CIRCLE THE CORRECT WORDS

Circle the correct word from the choices provided to complete these sentences.

15. When plasma volume increases to compensate for anemia, the blood viscosity (increases, decreases), which causes blood flow to be (sluggish, turbulent).

16. Defective DNA synthesis in bone marrow precursors usually creates erythrocytes that are (microcytic, macrocytic) and normochromic.

17. Folate deficiency anemia is associated with chronic malnourishment and chronic abuse of (cocaine, alcohol).

18. The incidence of iron deficiency anemia is (lowest, highest) in women during their reproductive years and (increases, decreases) after menopause.

19. People who are dehydrated after extensive diarrhea have (absolute, relative) polycythemia; people who have hypercapneic chronic obstructive pulmonary disease have (absolute, relative) polycythemia.

20. The most common causes of eosinophilia are (bacteria, parasites), toxic foreign particles, and (autoimmune, hypersensitivity) reactions.

21. Monocytosis occurs during the (early, late) phase of inflammation, whereas neutrophilia occurs during the (early, late) phase of inflammation.

22. All types of leukemias are characterized by uncontrolled (production, destruction) of white blood cells in the (blood, bone marrow) that thereby (decreases, increases) the amount and function of erythrocytes and platelets.

23. Although (leukopenia, leukocytosis) may occur pathologically or normally in response to physiologic stressors, (leukopenia, leukocytosis) occurs only pathologically.

24. In a leukemia or lymphoma that has the term *lymphoblastic* in its name, the malignant cells are (immature, well differentiated).

25. People who have thrombocythemia have a highest increased risk for (bleeding, clotting), although the other event also may occur.

CATEGORIZE ANEMIAS BY THE APPEARANCE OF THE ERYTHROCYTES

Write the appearance of the erythrocytes beside each type of anemia. Choices: normocytic-normochromic, macrocytic-normochromic, microcytic-hypochromic.

_____ 26. Iron deficiency anemia

_____ 27. Aplastic anemia

_____ 28. Pernicious anemia

_____ 29. Posthemorrhagic anemia

_____ 30. Folate deficiency anemia

DESCRIBE THE DIFFERENCES

Describe the difference between each pair of terms.

31. What is the difference between leukemias and lymphomas?

32. What is the difference between a lymphocytic leukemia and a myelogenous leukemia?

33. What is the difference between splenomegaly and hypersplenism?

34. What is the difference between the composition of arterial thrombi and venous thrombi?

MATCH THE ABNORMALITIES

Match the names of the abnormal items on the right with the descriptions on the left.

_____ 35. Autoantibody against plasma membrane components that causes hypercoagulability by binding to platelets and endothelial cells

A. Factor V Leiden

_____ 36. Abnormal antibody released by malignant plasma cells in multiple myeloma

B. Philadelphia chromosome

_____ 37. Genetic mutation that causes hypercoagulability by allowing activated clotting factor Va to remain longer in the blood

C. M protein

_____ 38. Genetic translocation between chromosomes 9 and 22 that creates a mutant protein implicated in CML and other types of leukemias

D. Antiphospholipid antibody

COMPLETE THE SENTENCES

Write one word in each blank to complete these sentences.

39. When describing the appearance of erythrocytes, terms that end with _____ refer to the hemoglobin content and terms that end with _____ refer to cell size.

40. Hereditary hemochromatosis is an autosomal _____ disorder that causes increased absorption of dietary _____.

41. Sideroblastic anemias are characterized by defective synthesis of _____.

42. Myelodysplastic syndrome involves defects in all lines of hematopoietic _____ cells; some people with this condition develop acute _____.

43. Serum ferritin levels are used to evaluate _____ status when diagnosing anemia.

44. Infectious mononucleosis is an acute infection of _____ lymphocytes commonly caused by Epstein-Barr _____; typical clinical manifestations are pharyngitis, fever, and cervical _____.

45. In Africa, _____ lymphoma, a rapidly growing _____ lymphocyte tumor in the _____ and facial bones of children is associated with Epstein-Barr _____.

46. AML stands for _____ _____ _____; CLL stands for _____ _____ _____.

47. Leukopenia creates increased risk for _____.

48. Hypercalcemia and bone lesions are characteristic of _____ _____ because the malignant cells reside in the bone marrow and not in the circulating blood.

49. Reed-Sternberg cells are the classic abnormal cells in _____ _____.

EXPLAIN THE PICTURES

Examine the pictures and answer the questions about them.

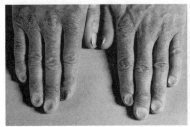 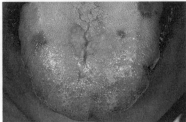

(From Hoffbrand AV, Pettit JE, Vyas P: *Color atlas of clinical hematology,* ed 4, London, 2009, Mosby.)

50. These pictures show the tongue and the fingernails from a person who has anemia. The tongue has lost papillae and looks fissured. What technical term describes it? _____

51. What technical term applies to the concave, brittle fingernails? _____

52. These pictures are characteristic of what type of anemia? _____

53. Would you expect this person to develop pallor or jaundice? Why?

54. Write a common scenario in which this type of anemia occurs.

TEACH PEOPLE ABOUT PATHOPHYSIOLOGY

Write your response to each situation in the space provided.

55. Mrs. Agee, who has polycythemia vera, says, "I thought red blood cells carry oxygen, not cause clotting. Why did I get a blood clot in my arm vein?"

56. Mrs. Montoya asks, "Why does anemia make me so tired?"

57. Mrs. Ferric was diagnosed recently with hereditary hemochromatosis. She says, "Tell me again how removing some of my blood regularly will help protect my liver."

58. "The doctor said they found Bence Jones proteins in my urine," said Mr. Thea. "What are Bence Jones proteins and why are they important?"

59. "I have multiple myeloma, which my oncologist says is malignant plasma cells," says Mr. Amon. "What are plasma cells? Do they have a normal function? What happens to that function when plasma cells become malignant?"

60. "Why is Knut so tired?" asks his wife. "He has ALL, but I thought leukemia is a problem with white blood cells. Knut is tired even when he does not have an infection."

61. "The doctor said my father is anemic," says Mrs. Fields, whose father has AML. "I think she should give him some iron tablets, like they gave me when I was anemic."

62. Mr. Squil has Hodgkin lymphoma. "When I get a sore throat, my neck nodes swell just a little and get tender," he says. "But with this Hodgkin lymphoma they swelled up a lot and were not tender at all. How can my lymph nodes swell so much but not be painful?"

63. "That medical student said my white cells are well differentiated," says Mr. Mihaly, who has CML. "What does that mean?"

64. Mr. Finn developed DIC while he was in a critical care unit with sepsis. Mrs. Finn says, "How can he be bleeding when he is making so many bad clots?"

65. Mrs. James says, "They told me I have ITP. I was so scared that I do not remember anything else. What is ITP? How does it make these red dots and purple blotches on my skin? Is it contagious?"

66. Mr. Drayson was admitted to the hospital with pneumonia. A nurse says, "He has von Willebrand disease also. What should I assess to see if it gets out of control?"

67. Mr. Vander Waal has thrombocytopenia from cancer chemotherapy. His son has immune thrombocytopenic purpura. "We have similar symptoms but different treatment," says Mr. Vander Waal. "Why?"

CLINICAL SCENARIO

Read the clinical scenario and answer the questions to explore your understanding of pernicious anemia.

Mrs. Swenson, age 64, was taken to an urgent care center after she fell getting off a bus. While her abrasions were being bandaged, she said, "My feet are numb and tingly, and I cannot always tell where they are." In answer to questions, she reported an 8-pound weight loss in the past 3 months, poor appetite, indigestion, sore tongue, and constant fatigue. Pallor was noted.

Laboratory Results

- Blood glucose, serum electrolytes, BUN, and creatinine normal

- Hemoglobin 8.0 g/dL (low) and hematocrit 32% (low)

- Macrocytic normochromic RBCs

Mrs. Swenson was directed to see her physician, who diagnosed pernicious anemia after additional testing.

68. What is the normal process of absorption of dietary vitamin B_{12}?

69. What caused Mrs. Swenson's pernicious anemia?

70. What is the technical description of erythrocyte size and color in pernicious anemia?

71. How are Mrs. Swenson's numbness and tingling related to pernicious anemia?

72. Mrs. Swenson is being treated with cobalamin (vitamin B$_{12}$) injections. After her blood vitamin B$_{12}$ level is brought back to normal, can her cobalamin be discontinued? Why or why not?

Chapter **21 Alterations of Hematologic Function**

22 Alterations of Hematologic Function in Children

MATCH THE DEFINITIONS

Match each word on the right with its definition on the left.

_____ 1. Breakdown of red blood cells

_____ 2. Formation of red blood cells

_____ 3. Presence of immature nucleated red blood cells in the blood

_____ 4. Normal enzyme that protects erythrocytes from oxidative damage

A. Erythroblastosis

B. Hemolysis

C. G6PD

D. Erythropoiesis

CIRCLE THE CORRECT WORDS

Circle the correct word from the choices provided to complete these sentences.

5. Iron deficiency anemia in children is highest before age (2, 14) because of an imbalance between dietary iron intake, the need for iron for normal (growth, G6PD function), and any occult blood loss.

6. Sickle cell disease is an autosomal (dominant, recessive) condition that is expressed in the (homozygous, heterozygous) form as sickle cell trait and in the (homozygous, heterozygous) form as sickle cell disease.

7. Sickle cell anemia often is detected at (birth, 6-12 months of age) because fetal hemoglobin (is, is not) affected by the genetic mutation.

8. If a child has sickle cell disease, factors that trigger sickling of erythrocytes include hypoxemia, (increased, decreased) pH of the blood, (fever, hypothermia), and (hypervolemia, hypovolemia).

9. When cells sickle in the microcirculation, they block blood flow, causing (painless, painful) infarction of local tissue.

10. Normally, four genes control synthesis of the hemoglobin (alpha, beta) chains and two genes control synthesis of the hemoglobin (alpha, beta) chains; this information is crucial to understanding the various forms of (sickle cell disease, thalassemia).

11. Normal adult hemoglobin is designated as hemoglobin (A, S).

DESCRIBE THE DIFFERENCES

Describe the difference between each pair of terms.

12. What is the difference between the chemical structures of hemoglobin A and hemoglobin S?

13. What is the genetic difference between sickle cell anemia and sickle cell trait?

COMPLETE THE SENTENCES

Write one word in each blank to complete these sentences.

14. Young children with sickle cell anemia may develop _____ crisis when large amounts of blood pool in the spleen and liver, potentially causing death from _____ _____.

15. Beta-thalassemia major also is called _____ anemia; the erythrocytes are unstable and prone to hemolysis because they have too many free hemoglobin _____ chains.

16. Children with hemophilia experience recurrent episodes of _____ and may develop limited mobility due to damage to _____ from some of these episodes.

17. The most common leukemia in children is acute _____ leukemia, which causes accumulation of _____ in bone marrow with resulting pallor, fatigue, purpura, bleeding, and fever.

18. Fever in acute leukemia is caused by _____ because of decreased neutrophils and by _____ from rapid growth of leukemic cells.

19. Hodgkin lymphoma is characterized by _____ enlargement of supraclavicular or cervical lymph nodes and has some association with Epstein-Barr _____.

20. Childhood non-Hodgkin lymphoma can arise from any _____ tissue and therefore has signs and symptoms that are specific to its location.

MATCH THE HEMOPHILIAS

Match the types of hemophilias on the right with the descriptions on the left.

_____ 21. Autosomal recessive factor XI deficiency   A. Hemophilia A

_____ 22. X-linked recessive factor VIII deficiency   B. Hemophilia B

_____ 23. X-linked recessive factor IX deficiency   C. Hemophilia C

TEACH PEOPLE ABOUT PATHOPHYSIOLOGY

Write your response to each situation in the space provided.

24. "What actually makes the red blood cells go into a sickle shape?" says Mrs. Han, a chemical engineer whose son has sickle cell anemia. "Give me the details!"

25. "Why did my nephew get yellow when he had a hemolytic crisis?" asks Mr. Tage. "I thought he would get pale from not having enough red blood cells."

CLINICAL SCENARIOS

Read the clinical scenarios and answer the questions to explore your understanding of hemolytic disease of the newborn.

Mrs. Scott received no prenatal care during her first pregnancy because of lack of money and transportation. Her neighbor helped her during childbirth, as she has helped many women in the area. The baby, Jacob, was healthy. Although Mrs. Scott has not been tested, she is Rh-negative. Mr. Scott and young Jacob are both Rh-positive. Mrs. Scott now is pregnant again.

26. Why is Mrs. Scott's fetus at risk for hemolytic disease of the newborn?

27. Why did Jacob, the first baby, not develop hemolytic disease of the newborn?

28. Ashley, Mrs. Scott's second baby, did develop hemolytic disease of the newborn. When baby Ashley was born, she was pale and her liver and spleen were somewhat enlarged. Why were these particular organs enlarged?

29. Baby Ashley was not jaundiced when she was born, but jaundice developed soon afterward. What caused her jaundice?

30. Why was baby Ashley not jaundiced when she was born?

31. What is kernicterus and why is it important in this situation?

Jim, age 10, developed unexplained multiple bruises on his torso. He did not tell anyone about them because he was afraid he would be in trouble. A few days later, his gym teacher noticed them when Jim's shirt flapped up during exercise. She reported a concern about child abuse to the authorities. After vigorous denial of abuse by Jim and his family and a visit to a physician, Jim was diagnosed with idiopathic thrombocytopenic purpura. His condition improved after 3 months of corticosteroid therapy.

32. The diagnostic blood work showed a low platelet count. What caused Jim's platelet count to be low?

33. Given the pathophysiology, what should the erythrocyte count have been? Why?

34. Why did Jim have multiple bruising?

23 Structure and Function of the Cardiovascular and Lymphatic Systems

MATCH THE DEFINITIONS

Match each word on the right with its definition on the left.

_____ 1. The pressure generated at the end of diastole

_____ 2. Volume of blood flowing into the systemic (or pulmonary) circuit in 1 minute

_____ 3. Ability to generate action potentials in a regular pattern

_____ 4. Ability to generate spontaneous depolarization to threshold potential

_____ 5. Resistance to ejection during systole

_____ 6. Ability of the heart muscle to shorten, generating force; change in developed tension at a given resting fiber length

A. Rhythmicity

B. Afterload

C. Preload

D. Contractility

E. Automaticity

F. Cardiac output

Name the structures below with their location in the picture, and then match their functions. The first one is completed as an example. Hint: Identify the structure first and then consider its function.

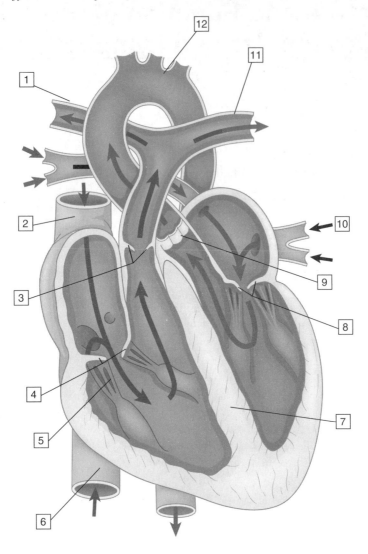

Name and Function of the Structure	Functions to Be Matched
7. Name: ___Right pulmonary artery___ Function: ___B___	A. Provides one-way flow of blood from the left ventricle into the aorta
8. Name: _____ Function: _____	B. Transports deoxygenated blood from the right ventricle to the right lung
9. Name: _____ Function: _____	C. Transports oxygenated blood from the left ventricle to the systemic circulation
10. Name: _____ Function: _____	D. Conveys deoxygenated blood from the head and upper extremities to the right atrium
11. Name: _____ Function: _____	E. Provides one-way flow of blood from the right ventricle into the pulmonary artery
12. Name: _____ Function: _____	F. Transports deoxygenated blood from the right ventricle to the left lung
13. Name: _____ Function: _____	G. Anchors the valve cusps to the papillary muscles to prevent valve prolapse
14. Name: _____ Function: _____	H. Conveys deoxygenated blood from the trunk and lower extremities to the right atrium
15. Name: _____ Function: _____	I. Transports oxygenated blood from the left lung to the left atrium
16. Name: _____ Function: _____	J. Provides one-way flow of blood from the left atrium into the left ventricle
17. Name: _____ Function: _____	K. Provides one-way flow of blood from the right atrium into the right ventricle
18. Name: _____ Function: _____	L. Separates the right and left ventricles

CIRCLE THE CORRECT WORDS

Circle the correct word from the choices provided to complete these sentences.

19. The right atrioventricular valve has (two, three) cusps and is called the (tricuspid, mitral) valve; the left atrioventricular valve has (two, three) cusps and is called the (tricuspid, mitral) valve.

20. Compared with skeletal muscle, cardiac muscle has (fewer, more) mitochondria and (fewer, more) T tubules.

21. Norepinephrine action on α-adrenergic receptors causes (vasoconstriction, vasodilation).

22. The myocardium normally extracts about (40%, 70%) of the oxygen from the coronary arteries; therefore it has a (small, large) oxygen reserve if myocardial oxygen demand increases.

23. Excitation-contraction coupling requires (calcium, magnesium).

24. At resting membrane potential, the inside of a myocardial cell is (less, more) negatively charged than the outside; when the myocardial cell depolarizes, the inside of the cell becomes (less, more) negatively charged.

25. Veins have (thinner, thicker) walls than arteries and are (less, more) compliant; valves are located in (both arteries and veins, veins only).

26. The tunica (media, intima) is the middle layer of blood vessels; it is composed of (endothelium and connective tissue, smooth muscle and elastic fibers).

27. Age-related changes in the cardiovascular system include (dilation, stiffening) of arterial walls.

SELECT THE FASTER ONE

Consider the pairs and select the one that is faster.

28. Which has a faster spontaneous depolarization rate: SA node or AV node?

29. Which has a faster spontaneous depolarization rate: AV node or Purkinje fibers?

30. Which causes a faster heart rate: sympathetic nerve firing or parasympathetic nerve firing?

31. Which is faster: blood flow in a capillary or blood flow in an arteriole?

CATEGORIZE THE EFFECTS

Write the type of initial effect beside each stimulus, assuming that no other factors also change. Choices for arterioles: vasoconstriction, vasodilation. *Choices for cardiac output or heart rate:* increase, decrease.

_____ 32. Norepinephrine effect on systemic arterioles

_____ 33. Epinephrine effect on systemic arterioles

_____ 34. Increased afterload effect on cardiac output

_____ 35. Physiologically increased preload effect on cardiac output

_____ 36. Large parasympathetic stimulation effect on cardiac output

_____ 37. Falling BP causing baroreceptor reflex effect on heart rate

_____ 38. Thyroid hormone effect on cardiac output

_____ 39. Nitric oxide local effect on arterioles

_____ 40. Endothelin local effect on arterioles

ORDER THE STEPS

Sequence the events that occur during the cardiac cycle.

41. Write the letters here in the correct order of the steps: _____
    A. Atrial pressure rises above ventricular pressure; mitral and tricuspid valves open; ventricles fill passively; pulmonary and aortic valves remain closed.
    B. Ventricular systole begins, and increasing intraventricular pressure closes the mitral and tricuspid valves; pulmonary and aortic valves remain closed.
    C. Ventricles relax and have little volume; pulmonary and aortic valves close; mitral and tricuspid valves remain closed; atria begin filling.
    D. Pulmonary and aortic valves are closed; mitral and tricuspid valves open; atria contract; ventricles are relaxed and they fill.
    E. Ventricular pressures exceed pulmonary artery and aortic pressures; pulmonary and aortic valves open; ventricular ejection occurs; mitral and tricuspid valves remain closed.

EXPLAIN THE PICTURE

Examine the electrocardiogram (ECG) and answer the questions about it.

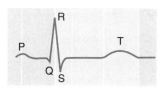

42. What electrical event occurs in the myocardium that generates the portion of the ECG marked P?

   _____

43. What do the atria do in response to this event?

   _____

44. Electrical signals are conducted through what parts of the heart during the PR interval?

   _____

45. What are the ventricles doing during the portion of the ECG that is shaded in the diagram (R through end of T wave)?

   _____

46. The mitral valve closes at approximately what location on the ECG? _____

47. Why is it important for the mitral and tricuspid valves to close at that time?

DESCRIBE THE DIFFERENCES

Describe the difference between each pair of terms.

48. What is the difference between the endocardium and the epicardium?

49. What is the difference between systole and diastole?

50. What is the difference between angiogenesis and arteriogenesis?

51. What is the difference between laminar flow and turbulent flow?

COMPLETE THE SENTENCES

Write one word in each blank to complete these sentences.

52. The aortic and pulmonary valves are the _____ valves, and they each have _____ cusps.

53. The _____ side of the heart is a high-pressure system, and the _____ side of the heart is a low-pressure system.

54. The _____ arteries bring oxygenated blood to the myocardium; venous blood from the myocardium empties into the _____ atrium.

55. Two important branches of the left coronary artery are the left _____ _____ artery and the _____ artery.

56. Parasympathetic nerves to the heart release the neurotransmitter _____, which binds to _____ receptors; sympathetic nerves to the heart release the neurotransmitter _____, which binds to _____ receptors.

57. As an action potential is transmitted through the T tubules, it triggers release of _____ from the sarco-plasmic reticulum.

58. An _____ disk is a thickened portion of the cardiac sarcolemma that enables rapid spread of depolarization between myofibrils.

59. The process of _____ enables an organ to regulate its blood flow by altering the resistance in its arterioles.

60. The right lymphatic duct and the _____ duct drain lymph into the _____ veins.

61. Small blood vessels that bring blood to the walls of large arteries are called vasa _____.

CALCULATE THE ANSWERS

Use the relevant portions of the information provided to calculate your answers.

Mrs. Ghent's blood pressure is 140/80 mm Hg, heart rate is 78 beats/min, stroke volume is 45 mL/beat, left ventricular end-diastolic volume is 75 mL/m^2, and respiratory rate is 18 breaths/min.

62. Her pulse pressure is _____.

63. Her mean arterial pressure is _____.

64. Her cardiac output is _____.

65. Her ejection fraction is _____.

SORT THE LAWS

Write the name of these laws beside their descriptions: Laplace law, Frank-Starling law of the heart, Poiseuille law.

_____ 66. Within limits, a greater end-diastolic volume will produce a greater contractile force during systole.

_____ 67. The amount of tension generated in a cardiac chamber or vessel to produce a given internal pressure varies directly with the radius and inversely with the wall thickness.

_____ 68. Blood flow is inversely related to resistance; resistance to blood flow is directly related to vessel length and blood viscosity and inversely related to the vessel radius to the fourth power.

TEACH PEOPLE ABOUT PHYSIOLOGY

Write your response to each situation in the space provided.

69. Kevin, age 17, says, "I am learning about the heart in high school. Why is the left ventricle muscle normally thicker than the right ventricle muscle? Why aren't they the same?"

70. A nurse who is new to the cardiac unit says, "I hear the cardiologists talking about blockage of the LAD. What are they discussing?"

71. An emergency department nurse says, "We always measure blood troponin levels in our suspected MI [myocardial infarction; heart attack] patients. I know that troponin normally is inside the myocardial cells, not in the blood. But what is the normal function of troponin?"

72. Mr. Pannopoulos asks, "When they transplant a heart, I know they cut the nerves. Do they have to put in a pacemaker to make the new heart beat after it is transplanted?"

24 Alterations of Cardiovascular Function

DECIPHER THE ACRONYMS

Use the clues to identify the acronyms and then write the words that each acronym represents.

Clues	Acronyms	Words Represented by the Acronyms
1. Clot formation in a large vein, usually in lower extremities		
2. Type of lipoprotein that migrates into arterial walls in atherosclerosis		
3. Heart attack that shows ST-segment elevation on ECG		
4. Atherosclerosis in the coronary arteries		
5. Heart disease caused by atherosclerosis in the coronary arteries		
6. Atherosclerosis in arteries that supply the extremities		
7. Mitral valve cusps billow backward into valve opening when valve should be closed		

MATCH THE DEFINITIONS

Match each word on the right with its definition on the left.

_____ 8. Distended and tortuous superficial veins in which blood has pooled

_____ 9. Sustained inadequate venous return caused by valvular damage

_____ 10. Ischemic pain in the lower extremities that occurs while walking but disappears when resting

_____ 11. Inflammatory disease of peripheral arteries that is associated with smoking

_____ 12. Vasospastic disorder of peripheral arteries in which episodes of ischemia and pallor are followed by rubor and paresthesias

_____ 13. Inflammation of the membranous sac that surrounds the heart

_____ 14. Compression of the heart by pericardial fluid

A. Intermittent claudication

B. Thromboangiitis obliterans

C. Raynaud phenomenon

D. Chronic venous insufficiency

E. Pericarditis

F. Tamponade

G. Varicose veins

CIRCLE THE CORRECT WORDS

Circle the correct word from the choices provided to complete these sentences.

15. Post-thrombotic syndrome is characterized by chronic persistent pain and (pallor and atrophy, edema and ulceration) of a limb that had deep venous thrombosis.

16. A major danger of deep venous thrombosis is development of (cerebral, pulmonary) thromboembolism; a danger of an arterial thrombus is development of (systemic, pulmonary) thromboembolism.

17. Superior vena cava syndrome occurs when a tumor or other mass (ruptures, compresses) the superior vena cava, causing (severe hypertension, venous distention) in the upper extremities and head.

18. Factors that cause primary hypertension increase peripheral vascular (responsiveness, resistance) and/or cause sustained (increase, decrease) in blood volume.

19. In hypertension, the pressure–natriuresis relationship shifts so that a hypertensive individual excretes (more, less) sodium in the urine.

20. People who have uncomplicated hypertension usually have (no, many) signs and symptoms in addition to their elevated blood pressure; treatment usually begins with (antihypertensive medications, lifestyle modifications).

21. The term *dissecting aneurysm* means that blood enters an artery wall and (runs between the layers of the wall, bursts through the wall and causes hemorrhage).

22. Risk for myocardial infarction increases with low blood levels of (LDL, HDL) and with high blood levels of (LDL, HDL).

23. Cardiac valve damage in rheumatic fever is caused by (group A β-hemolytic streptococci, an abnormal immune response); cardiac valve damage in infective endocarditis involves (streptococci or other organisms, an abnormal immune response).

24. Constrictive pericarditis is (an acute, a chronic) condition that can (compress, dilate) the heart.

EXPLAIN THE PICTURES

Examine the pictures and answer the questions about them.

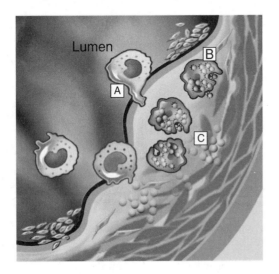
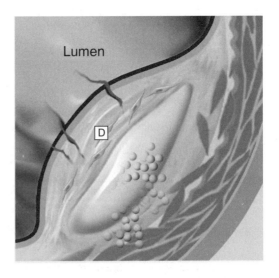

25. These pictures of artery walls show part of the disease process of _____

26. What is the monocyte labeled A doing? _____

27. What layer of the artery wall is the monocyte labeled A entering? _____

28. What are the abnormal globules that have accumulated in this layer of the artery wall? _____

29. What is the cell labeled B called? _____

30. What did the cell labeled B phagocytize that gave it its characteristic appearance? _____

31. The cell labeled C is a smooth muscle cell. What is it doing that is abnormal? _____

32. The cells labeled D are fibroblasts. What have they created? _____

33. Which picture illustrates a fibrous plaque? _____

34. What does the other picture illustrate? _____

CATEGORIZE THE CLINICAL MANIFESTATIONS

Write the type of heart failure that typically causes each sign or symptom. Choices: left heart failure, right heart failure.

_____ 35. Orthopnea

_____ 36. Ankle edema

_____ 37. Jugular venous distention

_____ 38. Dyspnea

_____ 39. Decreased urine output

_____ 40. Coughing pink frothy sputum

_____ 41. Crackles on auscultation

_____ 42. Hepatomegaly

DESCRIBE THE DIFFERENCES

Describe the difference between each pair of terms.

43. What is the difference between a thrombus and an embolus?

44. What is the difference between primary and secondary hypertension?

45. What is the difference between dilated and restrictive cardiomyopathy?

46. What is the difference between valvular stenosis and valvular regurgitation?

IDENTIFY THE RISK FACTORS

Use the clues to complete the list of risk factors for hypertension.

47.   H __ __ __ __ __ __
48.   __ __ __   Y __ __ __ __ __
49.   P __ __ __ __ __ __ __ __
50.   __ __   E
51.   R __ __ __ __
52. __ __ __ __ __   T __
53.   __ __ __ __   E __ __ __ __
54.   __   N __
55.   S __ __ __ __ __
56.   __   I __ __ __ __ __ __ __
57.   __ __ __   O __ __ __
58.   __   N __ __ __ __ __ __ __ __ __

Clues:

47. If this is positive in the family, risk increases.

48. Genetic character of hypertension.

49. Low dietary intake of this electrolyte is a risk factor.

50. As this increases, the risk increases.

51. Substance released by the kidneys that contributes to some cases of hypertension.

52. Modifiable risk factor estimated with BMI.

53. Low dietary intake of this electrolyte also is a risk factor.

54. Increased firing of this portion of the autonomic nervous system is a risk factor.

55. High dietary intake of this electrolyte is a risk factor.

56. Habitual use of these is a risk factor.

57. High intake of this recreational beverage is a risk factor.

58. With the word *glucose,* this is a major risk factor.

COMPLETE THE SENTENCES

Write one word in each blank to complete these sentences.

59. A clot in a blood vessel that breaks loose and circulates is called a _____.

60. Sluggish circulation from chronic venous insufficiency may cause a venous _____ ulcer.

61. Sustained hypertension causes left ventricular _____ and coronary atherosclerosis, thus increasing the risk for _____ _____.

62. Rapidly progressive hypertension with a diastolic pressure greater than 140 mm Hg is called _____ hypertension and can damage the _____.

63. Postural hypotension, also called _____ hypotension, is a systolic blood pressure decrease of at least _____ mm Hg or a diastolic blood pressure decrease of at least _____ mm Hg within 3 minutes of standing and is a significant risk factor for _____.

64. People who have subacute bacterial endocarditis are at risk for _____ embolism, whereas people who have trauma to long bones are at risk for _____ embolism.

65. The risk factors for peripheral arterial disease are the same as the risk factors for _____; the risk factors for coronary artery disease are the same as the risk factors for _____.

66. Clot formation at the site of rupture of an atherosclerotic plaque causes tissue _____, which leads to _____ if blood flow is not restored.

67. People who are obese have decreased levels of _____, an antiatherogenic adipokine.

68. Risk for myocardial infarction increases with factors that increase myocardial oxygen _____ or reduce myocardial oxygen _____.

69. Tissue healing after a myocardial infarction creates a noncontractile _____.

70. The ischemic injury from a sudden blockage of a coronary artery can be exacerbated by _____ injury when blood flow is restored.

71. Acute rheumatic fever is characterized by carditis, acute migratory _____, chorea, and _____ marginatum, which occur 1 to 5 weeks after streptococcal infection of the _____.

72. Prinzmetal angina, also called _____ angina, is caused by _____ of a coronary artery.

73. Angina caused by a clot temporarily occluding a coronary artery that resolves before necrosis occurs is called _____ angina.

MATCH THE CONSEQUENCES

Match the consequences on the right with the valve disorders on the left.

_____ 74. Aortic stenosis

_____ 75. Mitral regurgitation

_____ 76. Mitral stenosis

_____ 77. Tricuspid regurgitation

A. Right atrial and right ventricular dilation and hypertrophy

B. Left atrial hypertrophy and dilation

C. Left ventricular hypertrophy and dilation

D. Left atrial and left ventricular dilation and hypertrophy

TEACH PEOPLE ABOUT PATHOPHYSIOLOGY

Write your response to each situation in the space provided.

78. "Stress is all in your head!" says Mr. Weiss. "I do not want to take that stress management class! How can stress affect blood pressure?"

79. Mr. Evers has a newly diagnosed aortic aneurysm. "What is an aneurysm?" says Mrs. Evers. "And why do they want to operate to fix it? My husband feels fine!"

80. Mrs. Gao developed a deep venous thrombosis during a long car ride. "Tell me again those three big causes of leg clots," she says. "I want to avoid all of them in the future!"

81. "My uncle had a heart attack, and my father had a stroke," says Mr. Carradine. "My doctor said they were caused by the same thing, but I do not see how. Can you explain?"

82. "Why do I get so tired and faint when I try to exercise?" says Mr. Azul, who has mild aortic stenosis. "I am fine when I am not exercising."

83. "I heard the doctor tell the medical student that heart failure with reduced ejection fraction and heart failure with preserved ejection fraction are two kinds of heart failure," says Mr. Moon. "My doctor said I have heart failure with reduced ejection fraction, but I do not know what that means. Please explain."

84. Mr. Santos has left ventricular hypertrophy from hypertension. "How does that increase my risk of heart attack?" he says. "I think big strong muscles are a good thing!"

85. "My husband is in the emergency department, and they said he has acute coronary syndrome!" says Mrs. Gato. "Is that a heart attack?"

86. Mrs. Fewe was diagnosed with atrial fibrillation. "Oh, no! Grandma is dying! Call 911!" says Kendra, age 11, when she hears the diagnosis. "Fibrillation is an emergency!"

CLINICAL SCENARIOS

Read the clinical scenarios and answer the questions to explore your understanding of cardiac pathophysiology.

Mr. Kent, a 57-year-old nurse, developed crushing substernal chest pain with dyspnea, dizziness, and nausea while trying to lift a patient from a bed to a chair. In the emergency department, he states that his symptoms resolved as soon as he sat down to rest. Mr. Kent indicates that he has had similar episodes in the past, particularly when trying to do strenuous yard work. After an ECG and other tests, his diagnosis is stable angina.

87. What assessment questions should you ask Mr. Kent about his risk factors for coronary heart disease?

88. Why is it important to examine the appearance of Mr. Kent's lower extremities and palpate his pedal pulses?

89. Now that Mr. Kent's chest pain is completely resolved, what might his electrocardiogram show?

90. "I work pediatrics, not with adults," says Mr. Kent. "Remind me what stable angina is. It has been a long time since nursing school."

91. Mr. Kent says, "I seem to remember that some people have angina pain that is not in the chest. Is that correct?"

Chapter **24 Alterations of Cardiovascular Function**

92. "This is my wake-up call," says Mr. Kent. "I see that I need to take better care of myself. Tell me how eating less saturated fat will help. Maybe that will motivate me."

Mr. Williamson, age 81, had been feeling tired for several weeks. When he developed extreme shortness of breath, his wife took him to the emergency department. The emergency department personnel listened to his lungs, took a radiograph, and gave him an intravenous diuretic. He was admitted to the hospital with pulmonary edema from acute biventricular heart failure. After a few days, he was discharged from the hospital with various medications and instructions to eat a low-sodium diet and weigh himself every morning.

93. What fluid imbalance did Mr. Williamson have when he was taken to the emergency department? What parts of the case scenario provide the evidence for your answer?

94. What did the emergency department personnel hear when they listened to Mr. Williamson's lungs?

95. When Mr. Williamson was admitted to the hospital, what did assessment of his ankles most likely reveal? Why?

96. When Mr. Williamson was admitted to the hospital, what was the most likely character of his pulse?

97. Why was Mr. Williamson instructed to weigh himself every morning?

98. Why was a low-sodium diet prescribed for Mr. Williamson?

25 Alterations of Cardiovascular Function in Children

DECIPHER THE ACRONYMS

Use the clues to identify the acronyms and then write the words that each acronym represents.

Clues	Acronyms	Words Represented by the Acronyms
1. Congenital defect involving a hole in the septum between the two top cardiac chambers		
2. Congenital defect involving failure of the fetal blood vessel between the pulmonary artery and the aorta to close		
3. Congenital defect involving a hole in the septum between the two lower cardiac chambers		

CIRCLE THE CORRECT WORDS

Circle the correct word from the choices provided to complete these sentences.

4. Most congenital heart defects have begun to develop by the (8th, 18th) week of gestation.

5. Bluish coloration of mucous membranes and nail beds caused by presence of deoxygenated hemoglobin is called (hypoxemia, cyanosis).

6. Heart failure in children is (rarely, commonly) manifested by peripheral edema and neck vein distention in children.

7. The most common congenital heart defect is (atrial, ventricular) septal defect; many of these defects (will, will not) close spontaneously.

CHARACTERIZE THE CONGENITAL HEART DEFECTS

Write one letter and one number beside each picture of a congenital heart defect in the left column to indicate its name and the direction of blood shunt.

Picture of Congenital Heart Defect

Name of the Defect

Direction of the Blood Shunt
(Use each answer more than once)

A. Ventricular septal defect

B. Tricuspid atresia

C. Coarctation of the aorta

D. Atrial septal defect

E. Tetralogy of Fallot

F. Pulmonic stenosis

G. Patent ductus arteriosus

H. Aortic stenosis

1. Left to right

2. Right to left

3. No shunt

_____ 8.

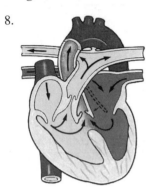

_____ 9.

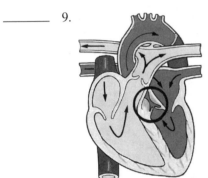

_____ 10.

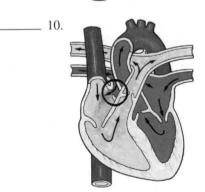

_____ 11.

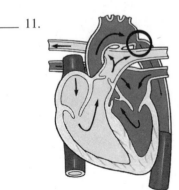

Chapter **25** Alterations of Cardiovascular Function in Children

_____ 12.

_____ 13.

_____ 14.

_____ 15.

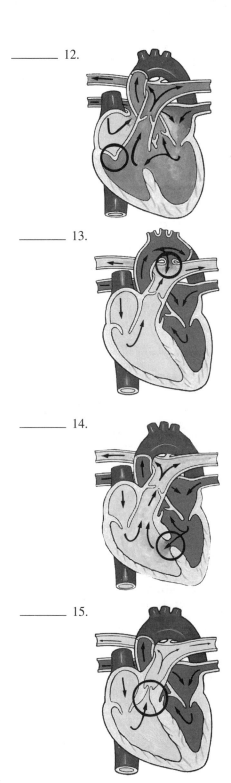

COMPLETE THE SENTENCES

Write one word in each blank to complete these sentences.

16. Blood flow through an abnormal cardiac opening always moves from an area of _____ pressure to an area of _____ pressure.

17. A congenital heart defect with a right-to-left shunt of blood is categorized as a _____ defect.

18. Failure of the endocardial cushions to fuse during fetal life causes an _____ canal defect and frequently occurs in children who have _____ syndrome.

19. Underdevelopment of the left side of the heart is termed _____ left heart syndrome.

20. With transposition of the great vessels, the aorta arises from the _____ ventricle, and the pulmonary artery arises from the _____ ventricle; unless additional defects are present, this defect is incompatible with _____ life.

21. The condition in which the pulmonary artery and the aorta are a single blood vessel is called _____ _____.

22. Young children who develop _____ disease have vasculitis of unknown cause and often develop aneurysms of their _____ arteries that may regress as the condition resolves.

23. Sustained hypertension in children often is associated with underlying _____ disease.

24. Children who are overweight often have _____.

TEACH PEOPLE ABOUT PATHOPHYSIOLOGY

Write your response to each situation in the space provided.

25. Mrs. Yu says, "The doctor said my baby has coarctation of his aorta. What is that? It sounds awful! And please tell me why the nurses keep taking blood pressure in my baby's leg. Is there something wrong with his leg too?"

26. Mrs. Quaid says, "The doctor said my baby has tetralogy of Fallot and drew me a picture of the four defects. But why does her little face turn that blue color when she cries? And why won't she nurse very long? Maybe she doesn't like me!"

27. Mr. Voll says, "The doctor said my baby has a patent ductus arteriosus. What is that? Isn't that ductus a normal thing? I remember that from going to the 'developing baby' class with my wife."

28. Mrs. Dee says, "The doctor said my baby has atrial septal defect. What is that? And then he said that my baby has a heart murmur! Does my baby have two heart problems?"

29. A nurse says, "Please explain why the signs and symptoms of a congenital heart defect that causes a right-to-left blood shunt are different from the signs and symptoms of a defect that causes a left-to-right blood shunt. I am having difficulty remembering that."

26 Structure and Function of the Pulmonary System

MATCH THE DEFINITIONS

Match each word on the right with its definition on the left.

_____ 1. Space between the lungs that contains the heart, great vessels, and esophagus

A. Surfactant

_____ 2. Substance secreted by type II alveolar cells that helps keep alveoli from collapsing

B. Hila

_____ 3. What goblet cells in the bronchi secrete

C. Elastin

_____ 4. A measure of distensibility

D. Carina

_____ 5. The structures that participate in gas exchange

E. Compliance

_____ 6. Membrane attached to the external side of the lungs

F. Acinus

_____ 7. Where the bronchi and pulmonary vessels enter the lungs

G. Pleura

_____ 8. Fibers that give lung tissue its elasticity

H. Mucus

_____ 9. Where the trachea divides into the two main bronchi

I. Mediastinum

ORDER THE STEPS

Beginning with the nose, sequence the structures through which air moves during inhalation.

10. Write the letters here in the correct order of the steps: _____
    A. Bronchioles
    B. Trachea
    C. Nasopharynx
    D. Bronchi
    E. Nose
    F. Respiratory bronchioles
    G. Larynx
    H. Alveoli
    I. Alveolar ducts

MATCH THE FUNCTIONS

Match the word on the right with its function on the left.

_____ 11. Prevent airway collapse during inhalation

A. Surfactant

_____ 12. Filter and humidify inspired air

B. Cartilage rings

_____ 13. Prevent lung collapse at end-exhalation

C. Pores of Kohn

_____ 14. Allow pressure to equalize between adjacent alveoli

D. Nasopharynx

CIRCLE THE CORRECT WORDS

Circle the correct word from the choices provided to complete these sentences.

15. The left lobe of the lung has (two, three) lobes; the right lobe of the lung has (two, three) lobes.

16. The pulmonary circulation has (lower, higher) pressure and resistance than the systemic circulation.

17. Pulmonary (arteries, veins) are spaced randomly throughout the lungs, but the pulmonary (arteries, veins) run beside the branches of the airways.

18. Pulmonary veins carry (oxygenated, deoxygenated) blood and are attached to the (right, left) atrium.

19. The most effective way to measure the adequacy of alveolar ventilation is to measure (ventilatory effort, $Paco_2$).

20. The neurons that control respiration are located in the (basal ganglia, brainstem).

21. Parasympathetic stimulation causes airways to (dilate, constrict); sympathetic stimulation causes airways to (dilate, constrict).

22. The (internal, external) intercostal muscles are active during vigorous inspiration.

23. In a person at sea level breathing through the nose, the gas that reaches the lungs is fully saturated with (water vapor, carbon dioxide); the partial pressure of oxygen in that case is calculated by ($[(760 \times 0.209) - 47]$, $[(760 - 47) \times 0.209]$).

24. The shift in the oxyhemoglobin dissociation curve caused by alterations in pH and $Paco_2$ is called the (Haldane, Bohr) effect.

EXPLAIN THE PICTURE

Examine the picture and answer the questions about it.

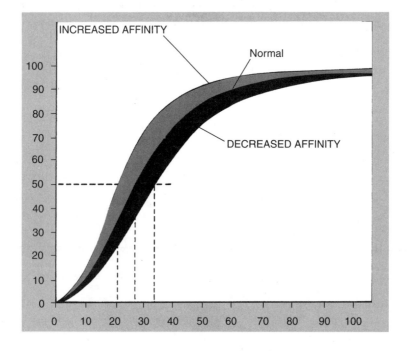

Chapter **26** **Structure and Function of the Pulmonary System**

25. This picture shows an oxyhemoglobin dissociation curve. What parameter is measured on the horizontal axis? _____

26. What parameter is measured on the vertical axis? _____

27. Which chemoreceptors, central or peripheral, will respond if the parameter measured on the horizontal axis falls to 55 mm Hg? _____

28. Which side (left or right) of the curve represents the situation of blood in the lungs? _____ In what way is that beneficial? _____

29. Which side (left or right) of the curve represents the situation of blood in the tissues? _____ In what way is that beneficial? _____

30. List three factors that cause this shift to occur in the tissues. _____

_____

31. Which way does the curve shift when a patient is hypothermic? _____

DESCRIBE THE DIFFERENCES

Describe the difference between each pair of terms.

32. What is the difference between a terminal bronchiole and a respiratory bronchiole?

33. What is the difference between type I and type II alveolar cells?

34. What is the difference between the visceral pleura and the parietal pleura?

35. What is the difference between Pao_2 and Pao_2?

36. What is the difference between ventilation and respiration?

COMPLETE THE SENTENCES

Write one word in each blank to complete these sentences.

37. The nasopharynx and oropharynx are the _____ airway.

38. The mononuclear phagocytic cells in the lungs are called alveolar _____.

39. The structures that comprise the acinus are the _____ bronchioles, the _____ ducts, and the _____.

40. Gas exchange occurs across the _____ membrane.

41. A person with a respiratory rate of 12 breaths per minute and a minute volume of 6.0 L per minute has a tidal volume of _____ mL.

42. Receptors in the conducting airways that initiate the cough reflex in response to inhaled dust are called _____ receptors.

43. During inspiration, the diaphragm moves _____, which _____ the volume of the thoracic cavity, creating _____ pressure that draws air into the lungs.

44. Normal lung tissue returns to its resting state after inspiration because it has _____ recoil.

45. Lungs that are fibrotic and stiff have _____ compliance, which _____ the work of breathing, thus _____ oxygen demand.

46. The V/Q ratio of a normal upright lung is _____, which indicates that ventilation is _____ than perfusion.

47. Blood gas analysis in a healthy older adult is most likely to show a decrease in _____.

MATCH THE ZONES

Match the lung zones of an upright lung on the right with the descriptions on the left.

_____ 48. Perfusion is greater than ventilation because pulmonary arterial and venous pressures are greater than alveolar pressure.

A. Zone I

_____ 49. Perfusion is happening but is not maximum because pulmonary arterial and venous pressures are opposed by alveolar pressure.

B. Zone II

_____ 50. No perfusion occurs because alveolar pressure is greater than pulmonary arterial and venous pressures.

C. Zone III

TEACH PEOPLE ABOUT PHYSIOLOGY

Write your response to each situation in the space provided.

51. "I read that smoking makes the cilia in airways not work well," says Mr. Lewis. "What do those cilia do when they ARE working?"

52. "Please explain why the blood in the left heart in a healthy adult is not quite 100% oxygenated," says a nurse. "After blood goes through the lungs, it should be fully oxygenated."

53. "I learned that pulmonary arterioles constrict when alveolar partial pressure of oxygen is low in a portion of a lung," says a physiology student. "In what way is that beneficial?"

54. "My respiratory patient has hypoxemia but his Pa_{CO_2} is normal," says a nurse. "How is that possible?"

27 Alterations of Pulmonary Function

MATCH THE DEFINITIONS

Match each word on the right with its definition on the left.

_____ 1. Presence of pus in the pleural cavity

_____ 2. Collapse of alveoli

_____ 3. Bluish discoloration of the skin caused by desaturation of hemoglobin

_____ 4. Pao$_2$ below normal

_____ 5. Coughing up bloody mucus

_____ 6. Passage of fluid and/or solid particles into the lungs

A. Cyanosis

B. Hypoxemia

C. Hemoptysis

D. Empyema

E. Atelectasis

F. Aspiration

CIRCLE THE CORRECT WORDS

Circle the correct word from the choices provided to complete these sentences.

7. Hyperventilation causes decreased (Paco$_2$, Pao$_2$).

8. Presence of fluid in the pleural space is called pleural (edema, effusion).

9. Severe kyphoscoliosis causes (increased, decreased) chest wall compliance.

10. People who have difficulty (coughing, swallowing) have increased risk for aspiration; aspiration of gastric acid is most likely to cause (bronchiolitis, pneumonitis).

11. A person who has pulmonary edema will have (resonance, dullness) to percussion over the lung bases, inspiratory (wheezing, crackles), and with severe pulmonary edema, (foul-smelling, pink frothy) sputum.

12. Processes that increase capillary permeability can cause (exudative, transudative) pleural effusion, but processes that increase capillary hydrostatic pressure can cause (exudative, transudative) pleural effusion.

13. Clinical manifestations of bronchiolitis include tachypnea, (productive, nonproductive) cough, use of accessory muscles, (low-grade, high) fever, and hypoxemia.

14. Silicosis is a(n) (obstructive, restrictive) respiratory disease; asthma is a(n) (obstructive, restrictive) respiratory disease.

15. People who have obstructive respiratory disorders have the most difficulty with (inspiration, expiration).

16. Clubbing of the fingers is a response to (acute, chronic) hypoxemia.

17. The most common cause of lung cancer in the United States is (poor nutrition, cigarette smoking); early lung cancer has (vague, obvious) signs and symptoms.

CATEGORIZE THE CAUSES

Write the ventilation problem beside each cause. Choices: hypoventilation, hyperventilation.

_____ 18. Head injury

_____ 19. Airway obstruction

_____ 20. Reduced firing of neurons to respiratory muscles

_____ 21. Anxiety

_____ 22. Respiratory muscle weakness

_____ 23. Response to severe hypoxemia

_____ 24. Reduced compliance of chest wall

ORDER THE STEPS

Sequence the events that occur during the development of acute respiratory distress syndrome.

25. Write the letters here in the correct order of the steps: _____
    A. Neutrophils release inflammatory mediators.
    B. Pulmonary edema occurs from hemorrhagic exudate.
    C. Neutrophils, macrophages, and platelets accumulate in the lungs.
    D. Pneumonia or an other condition causes acute lung injury.
    E. Fibrosis destroys alveoli and bronchioles.
    F. Cell damage disrupts alveolocapillary membrane.
    G. Acute respiratory failure occurs with hypoxemia, hypercapnia, and acidosis.
    H. Fibroblasts and other lung cells proliferate and form membranes from granulation tissue.

EXPLAIN THE PICTURE

Examine the picture and answer the questions about it.

26. This picture shows a portion of the pathophysiology of an acute
    episode of _____

27. From the information in the picture, was this the first time the individual was exposed to the antigen? Explain your answer.

28. What is the source of the IgE that binds to mast cells?

29. What happens when antigen binds to the IgE located on the mast cells? Why is that important?

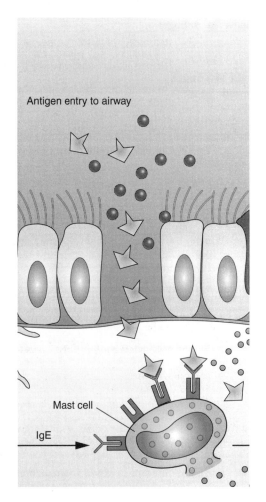

DESCRIBE THE DIFFERENCES

Describe the difference between each pair of terms.

30. What is the difference between dyspnea and orthopnea?

31. What is the difference between absorption atelectasis and compression atelectasis?

32. What is the difference between communicating pneumothorax and tension pneumothorax?

Chapter **27** **Alterations of Pulmonary Function**

MATCH THE BREATHING PATTERNS

Match the breathing patterns on the right with the descriptions on the left.

_____ 33. Alternating periods of deep and shallow breathing with apnea episodes

_____ 34. Increased ventilatory rate, small tidal volume

_____ 35. Rhythmic and effortless with normal tidal volume

_____ 36. Irregular, quick inspirations with an expiratory pause

_____ 37. Increased ventilatory rate, small tidal volume, increased effort, prolonged expiration, wheezing

_____ 38. Increased ventilatory rate, very large tidal volume, no expiratory pause

A. Kussmaul

B. Gasping

C. Cheyne-Stokes

D. Eupnea

E. Restricted

F. Obstructed

COMPLETE THE SENTENCES

Write one word in each blank to complete these sentences.

39. Waking up with dyspnea during the night and needing to sit upright or stand to breathe is called _____ _____ _____.

40. Rib fractures that disrupt the mechanics of breathing can cause a portion of the chest wall to collapse _____ during inspiration, an acute condition known as _____ chest.

41. A person who has pneumothorax has _____ in the pleural space.

42. A person who has _____ has persistent abnormal dilations of the bronchi and a chronic cough that produces large amounts of purulent _____.

43. Pulmonary fibrosis is an excessive amount of _____ tissue in the lungs and causes _____ lung compliance.

44. In asthma, long-term airway damage that is irreversible is known as airway _____.

45. During an acute asthma episode, inflammatory mediators cause inflammation, hypersecretion of _____, and bronchial smooth muscle _____.

46. An asthma episode that does not resolve with usual treatment is called _____ _____.

47. Genetic deficiency of _____ _____ causes early-onset emphysema because this enzyme normally inhibits the action of _____ _____ that can destroy lung tissue.

48. The two disorders known as COPD are emphysema and _____ _____ this latter condition is characterized by persistent hypersecretion of _____ and chronic _____ cough.

49. Clinical manifestations of emphysema include _____ chest and _____ on exertion and eventually at rest.

50. Cor pulmonale is _____ ventricular enlargement caused by chronic pulmonary _____.

51. Laryngeal cancer is characterized by progressive _____.

52. Primary lung cancer arising from cells that line the airways is called _____ _____; small cell

   carcinoma in the lung often produces tumor-derived _____.

TEACH PEOPLE ABOUT PATHOPHYSIOLOGY

Write your response to each situation in the space provided.

53. "Why does Grandpa have to breathe so hard?" says Ben, age 14, whose grandfather has emphysema.

54. "My uncle has ARDS," says Simon, age 10. "What does ARDS mean and what is wrong with him?"

55. "My cousin's arm tested positive for tuberculosis, but he does not feel sick and his x-ray is good," says Marsh, age 11. "When will he start coughing up blood like in the movies?"

56. "How did working in the coal mine make grandpa have trouble breathing?" says Jonah, age 8, whose grandfather has pulmonary fibrosis.

57. Mr. Rudofski says, "My grandfather was a sand blaster and got pulmonary fibrosis from years of exposure to silica. My uncle was a rare book librarian and got pulmonary fibrosis from years of exposure to book mold. They both had pulmonary fibrosis, with similar symptoms, but the doctors called one condition a 'pneumoconiosis' and the other a 'hypersensitivity pneumonitis.' Please explain why."

58. "My husband had difficulty breathing; at the emergency department they said he had water in his lungs because the left side of his heart was not working properly," says Mrs. Hoody. "How can a problem with the heart cause water in the lungs?"

Chapter **27** **Alterations of Pulmonary Function**

Read the clinical scenarios and answer the questions to explore your understanding of respiratory disorders.

Mrs. Beeson, age 64, who has a long history of smoking, developed pleuritic chest pain in the right side of her chest. She also has a high fever, dyspnea, and a cough. On examination, she has absent breath sounds on the right and a pleural friction rub.

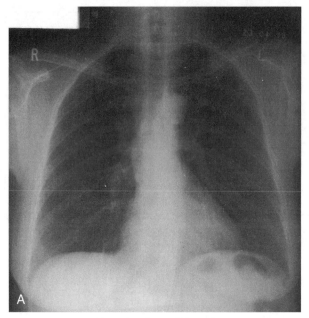

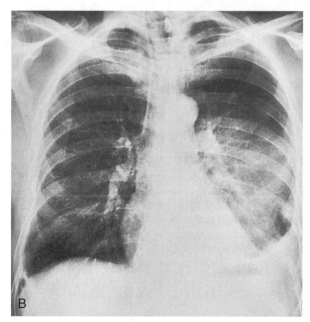

| Normal radiograph (x-ray) | Mrs. Beeson's radiograph |

(Courtesy) **A,** Davies A, Moores C: *The respiratory system,* ed 2, Philadelphia, 2010, Churchill Livingstone. **B,** Hansell DM, et al: *Imaging of disease of the chest,* ed 5, Philadelphia, 2010, Mosby.

Mrs. Beeson's radiograph shows a dense white collection of fluid at the base of the left lung, where it obscures the left diaphragm and much of the lower left lung. Thoracentesis reveals numerous white blood cells and bacteria in her pleural fluid. Ms. Beeson's diagnosis is empyema.

59. What is empyema?

60. Where does empyema fluid usually originate?

61. Why does Mrs. Beeson experience dyspnea?

Mrs. Goh, age 46, emigrated from Southeast Asia 25 years ago. She is admitted to the hospital with low-grade fever, shortness of breath, and a cough producing discolored sputum. Further evaluation reveals that she has had an unintentional weight loss of 15 pounds in the past 4 months. Examination of her sputum is positive for *Mycobacterium tuberculosis.* Her diagnosis is active tuberculosis (TB) disease.

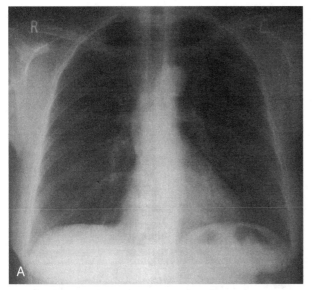

Normal radiograph (x-ray)

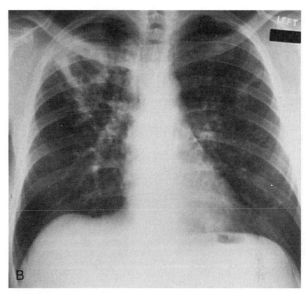

Mrs. Goh's radiograph

(Courtesy) **A,** Davies A, Moores C: *The respiratory system,* ed 2, Philadelphia, 2010, Churchill Livingstone. **B,** Mason RJ, Broaddus VC, Murray JF: *Murray and Nadel's textbook of respiratory medicine,* ed 4, Philadelphia, 2010, Saunders.

Mrs. Goh's radiograph shows cavitary disease in the right lung. Mrs. Goh was infected with the TB bacillus when she lived in Southeast Asia. Until several months ago, the TB bacilli were sequestered in a tubercle.

62. How is tuberculosis transmitted?

63. What is a tubercle?

64. When the TB bacilli were sequestered in the tubercle, did Mrs. Goh have a positive tuberculin test? Explain your answer.

65. Mrs. Goh's TB infection reactivated. Why might this have occurred after at least 25 years?

66. In addition to the radiograph and sputum findings, what signs and symptoms of active TB disease that Mrs. Goh had are mentioned in the case scenario?

Mrs. Yarborough, age 47, who smokes a pack of cigarettes per day, has developed fever, chills, dyspnea, and a cough productive of yellow-green sputum. Her body temperature is 101.3° F (38.5° C). She has tachypnea, tachycardia, and inspiratory crackles auscultated over her right upper and lower lung. Sputum stain reveals numerous white blood cells and bacteria.

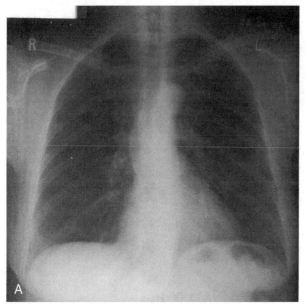

Normal radiograph (x-ray)

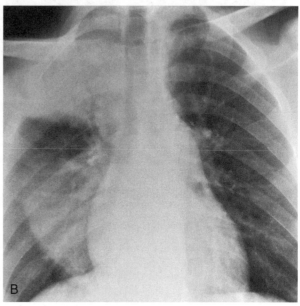

Mrs. Yarborough's radiograph

(Courtesy) **A,** Davies A, Moores C: *The respiratory system,* ed 2, Philadelphia, 2010, Churchill Livingstone. **B,** Lafleur Brooks M: *Exploring medical language,* ed 7, St Louis, 2009, Mosby.

67. Does Mrs. Yarborough have bacterial or viral pneumonia? Explain your answer.

68. What is the pathophysiology of Mrs. Yarborough's illness?

69. What will clear the consolidated exudate from her alveoli as she recovers?

70. Why is smoking cessation important for Mrs. Yarborough to help prevent another episode of pneumonia?

Ms. Kelly Silber, age 24, was admitted yesterday for a femur fracture from a skiing accident. She develops sudden dyspnea and pain in the left side of her chest that is worse with breathing. Assessment reveals tachypnea, tachycardia, and some slight crackles in the lower left lung. Ms. Silber's serum D-dimer is elevated. Spiral CT arteriography confirmed her diagnosis of pulmonary embolism.

71. How did Ms. Silber develop a pulmonary embolism?

72. How does a large pulmonary embolism cause V/Q mismatch?

73. Ms. Silber asks, "What is the connection between my broken leg and this breathing problem?" Respond as if speaking directly to Ms. Silber.

28 Alterations of Pulmonary Function in Children

MATCH THE DEFINITIONS

Match each word on the right with its definition on the left.

_____ 1. Infection and inflammation in the terminal airways and alveoli

_____ 2. Acute laryngotracheitis, seen in young children

_____ 3. Harsh vibratory sound with variable pitch caused by turbulent airflow through a partially obstructed upper airway

_____ 4. Viral lower respiratory tract infection, seen in infants

A. Stridor

B. Bronchiolitis

C. Croup

D. Pneumonia

CIRCLE THE CORRECT WORDS

Circle the correct word from the choices provided to complete these sentences.

5. The cough associated with croup is a (productive, barking) cough.

6. Acute epiglottitis classically is a (viral, bacterial) infection and most commonly occurs in children aged (2 to 7, 7 to 12) years.

7. Peritonsillar abscess usually is (unilateral, bilateral) and is a complication of (tonsillitis, infectious mononucleosis).

8. Pneumonia in young children most commonly is a (viral, bacterial) infection.

9. Pneumonia caused by *Mycoplasma* is known as (bacterial, atypical) pneumonia and usually is (not, very) clinically severe.

10. ARDS (precedes, follows) ALI and is characterized by (progressive, recurrent) respiratory distress and severe (hypercarbia, hypoxemia).

CATEGORIZE THE RESPIRATORY DISORDERS

Write the type of disorder beside each name. Choices: upper airway infection, lower airway infection.

_____ 11. Tonsillitis

_____ 12. Bronchiolitis

_____ 13. Bacterial tracheitis

_____ 14. Pneumonia

_____ 15. Retropharyngeal abscess

_____ 16. Peritonsillar abscess

EXPLAIN THE PICTURE

Examine the picture and answer the questions about it.

17. This picture shows areas associated with specific clinical manifestations in a child with upper airway obstruction. Which letter on the picture denotes the area where an obstruction will cause a weak cry or hoarse voice? _____

18. Which letter denotes the area where an obstruction will cause snoring? _____

19. What is the significance of the area marked E? _____

20. What sound is associated with obstruction in areas B and C? _____

21. If obstruction in area B or C produces the same sound, why are they marked as different areas? _____

22. Obstructive sleep apnea is associated with sounds made in which _____

COMPLETE THE SENTENCES

Write one word in each blank to complete these sentences.

23. The acronym RDS stands for _____ _____ _____

24. Acute laryngotracheobronchitis, *commonly called* _____, usually is caused by a _____ that causes _____ edema.

25. The most common predisposing factor for childhood obstructive sleep apnea is _____ hypertrophy.

26. Respiratory distress syndrome of the newborn is caused by _____ deficiency; fibrin deposits in the alveoli create the appearance of _____ membranes, which gave the condition its previous name.

27. Chronic lung disease of prematurity, also called _____ _____, is associated with arrested lung _____.

28. Bronchiolitis is most commonly caused by _____ _____ _____; symptoms include initial _____, cough, and _____ respiratory rate.

29. Meconium aspiration causes aspiration _____.

30. The _____ hypothesis attempts to explain the increased incidence of asthma in developed cultures.

TEACH PEOPLE ABOUT PATHOPHYSIOLOGY

Write your response to each situation in the space provided.

31. "What is croup?" asks Sandi, age 10. "My little brother had croup and it was scary! Will I get it?"

32. Mrs. Jones took her son Jason, age 9, to a nurse practitioner because his teacher reported that Jason keeps falling asleep in school and his grades are poor. "The nurse practitioner asked if Jason snores," she said. "Why did she ask that?"

33. "My cousin's baby died of SIDS," says Mrs. Bush, whose son Howie is 18 months old. "Now I set my alarm every 2 hours during the night to be sure that Howie is breathing."

34. Kevin, age 14, aspirated a chunk of hot dog during a hot dog eating contest. He choked and wheezed at the time but soon recovered and kept gobbling hot dogs until the contest concluded. Several days later, he began wheezing again and his mother took him to a physician assistant, who discovered the aspirated item. "I am fine!" says Kevin. "Why do you have to put that tube down my throat to remove that piece of hot dog? Won't it eventually dissolve anyway?"

35. Molly, age 6, developed acute cough, wheeze, and dyspnea after playing with her cousin's dog. "Why did she get asthma from the dog?" asks her brother, age 10. "Was it dog germs? I play with the dog all the time but I do not get asthma."

CLINICAL SCENARIOS

Read the clinical scenarios and answer the questions to explore your understanding of acute epiglottitis and cystic fibrosis.

Darrell, age 4, had difficulty breathing and was drooling. His mother rushed him to the emergency department. Based on the following assessment, the admitting nurse immediately called an anesthesiologist, who intubated Darrell.

Objective Findings

- Tripod posture

- Drooling

- Voice muffled

- Inspiratory stridor

- Obvious use of accessory muscles during inspiration

- Temperature 102° F (38.9° C) (tympanic)

Subjective Findings

- Child reports sore throat

- Mother reports sudden onset

Darrell's diagnosis is acute epiglottitis. On follow-up, it was determined that Darrell had not received any immunizations.

36. The admitting nurse did not examine Darrell's throat. Was this an error on her part?

37. Why was Darrell drooling?

38. What caused Darrell's stridor?

39. Explain to Darrell's mother what the epiglottis is and what epiglottitis means.

40. Why was Darrell given intravenous antibiotics instead of oral ones?

41. What is the usual clinical course of acute epiglottitis that is treated with intubation and antibiotics?

Wilson, age 15, has cystic fibrosis (CF) that was diagnosed when he was an infant. He is thin, small for his age, and has recurrent respiratory infections.

42. Wilson says, "If I inherited CF from my parents, why don't they have CF?"

43. What is CFTCR and why is it important in CF?

44. Why does Wilson have recurrent respiratory infections?

45. What is the role of neutrophils in CF?

46. In what way is biofilm formation important in CF?

47. Examination of Wilson's hands is likely to reveal what findings?

48. How does the pathophysiology of CF contribute to Wilson being thin and small for his age?

29 Structure and Function of the Renal and Urologic Systems

MATCH THE DEFINITIONS

Match each word on the right with its definition on the left.

_____ 1. The process of urination

_____ 2. Chamber of the kidney through which urine passes into the renal pelvis

_____ 3. The bladder wall muscle

_____ 4. Cone-shaped section of the renal medulla that contains loops of Henle and collecting ducts

_____ 5. The area of the bladder between the openings of the ureters and the urethra

_____ 6. The area of the kidney where the ureter exits and blood vessels enter and exit

A. Detrusor

B. Trigone

C. Micturition

D. Calyx

E. Hilum

F. Pyramid

CIRCLE THE CORRECT WORDS

Circle the correct word from the choices provided to complete these sentences.

7. All of the glomeruli are located in the renal (medulla, cortex).

8. The (internal, external) urethral sphincter is under voluntary control.

9. Urea is a product of (carbohydrate, protein) metabolism; recycling of urea within the renal medulla is necessary to (concentrate; filter) urine.

10. Elimination of a substance in the urine is called (secretion, excretion).

11. The amount of plasma filtered per unit time is the (glomerular filtration rate, filtration fraction).

12. Natriuretic peptides (increase, decrease) renal excretion of sodium and water; ADH (increases, decreases) renal excretion of water, which (increases, decreases) urine specific gravity.

13. Blood entering the peritubular capillaries has (low, high) hydrostatic pressure and (low, high) oncotic pressure, which facilitates (secretion, reabsorption) of fluid from the proximal convoluted tubules.

14. Tamm-Horsfall protein, also known as (nephrin, uromodulin), is produced in the (proximal, distal) nephron segments and protects against (bacteria, viruses).

15. The concentration gradient of the renal interstitium (decreases, increases) from the cortex to the tip of the medulla; this gradient is necessary in order to (dilute, concentrate) the urine.

16. The countercurrent exchange system operates because fluid flows in opposite directions through the two segments of the (loop of Henle, vasa recta) and the gradient is maintained by the (loop of Henle, vasa recta).

17. The kidneys (activate, inactivate) vitamin D, a process that is stimulated by (calcitonin, parathyroid hormone).

18. Creatinine or cystatin C clearance is used to estimate (renal blood flow, glomerular filtration rate); para-aminohippuric acid clearance is used to estimate (renal blood flow, glomerular filtration rate).

LOCATE THE STRUCTURES

Write the type of anatomic location in the kidney beside each structure. Choices: renal cortex, renal medulla.

_____ 19. Glomeruli

_____ 20. Collecting ducts

_____ 21. Most of the proximal tubules

_____ 22. Glomerular capillaries

_____ 23. Most of the distal tubules

_____ 24. Pyramids

_____ 25. Most of the vasa recta

_____ 26. Renal corpuscles

_____ 27. Interlobular arteries

_____ 28. Afferent arterioles

ORDER THE STEPS

Sequence the structures through which fluid flows, starting in the glomerulus and ending as urine in the bladder.

29. Write the letters here in the correct order of the steps: _____
    A. Glomerular capillaries
    B. Proximal convoluted tubule
    C. Bladder
    D. Renal pelvis
    E. Filtration slits
    F. Loop of Henle
    G. Bowman's capsule
    H. Distal convoluted tubule
    I. Ureter
    J. Collecting duct

MATCH THE FUNCTIONS

Match the portion of the nephron on the right with its function on the left.

_____ 30. Reabsorption of large amounts of sodium, water, glucose, amino acids; net reabsorption of bicarbonate; secretion of H^+, organic acids, and many medications

A. Glomerulus

_____ 31. Reabsorption of sodium, chloride, and potassium but not much water

B. Distal tubule and collecting duct

_____ 32. Secretion of potassium, ammonia, and H^+; site of action of aldosterone and ADH

C. Proximal tubule

_____ 33. Filtration

D. Descending limb of loop of Henle

_____ 34. Reabsorption of water

E. Thick ascending limb of loop of Henle

EXPLAIN THE PICTURE

Examine the picture and answer the questions about it.

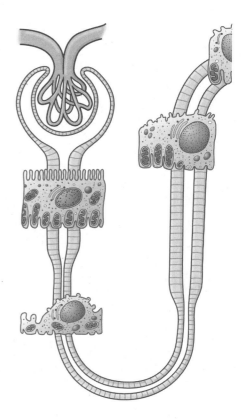

35. The first cell pictured below Bowman's capsule is in what portion of the nephron?

    _____

36. What is the significance of the large number of mitochondria in this cell?

37. What is the significance of the microvilli on the luminal surface of this cell?

38. Compare the cells pictured on the descending limb of the loop of Henle and the thick ascending limb. Which one has larger mitochondria and thus is more suited for active transport of solutes?

    _____

Chapter **29** **Structure and Function of the Renal and Urologic Systems**

MATCH THE MECHANISMS

Match the mechanism on the right with its description on the left.

_____ 39. A process that regulates sodium and water balance by reabsorption of a constant fraction of the sodium load filtered at the glomerulus.

_____ 40. A process that regulates renal blood flow and glomerular filtration rate to keep them constant by altering the amount of vasoconstriction of afferent arterioles in response to changes in their circumference.

_____ 41. A process that regulates renal blood flow and glomerular filtration rate to keep them constant by altering the amount of vasoconstriction of afferent arterioles in response to changes in the concentration of filtered sodium.

A. Tubuloglomerular feedback

B. Glomerulotubular balance

C. Myogenic mechanism

DESCRIBE THE DIFFERENCES

Describe the difference between each pair of terms.

42. What is the difference between urethra and ureter?

43. What is the difference between the principal cells and the intercalated cells in the collecting duct?

44. What is the difference between tubular secretion and tubular reabsorption?

COMPLETE THE SENTENCES

Write one word in each blank to complete these sentences.

45. The epithelial cells of the proximal convoluted tubule are the only renal tubular cells that have _____.

46. The _____ is the functional unit of the kidney; the _____ ones are highly important for concentrating urine.

47. Glomerular capillary blood flow is regulated in part by the contractile _____ cells and by vasoactive substances secreted by the endothelium.

48. The filtration fraction is the ratio of the glomerular filtration rate to _____ _____ _____.

49. Renal arterioles are innervated by _____ nerves; increased firing of these nerves causes the arterioles to

_____.

50. Net glomerular filtration pressure is the sum of the forces that _____ filtration minus the forces that

_____ filtration.

51. The renal hormone _____ degrades catecholamines.

52. In response to hypoxia, the kidneys secrete _____, which circulates to bone marrow and stimulates

_____.

53. The term _____ refers to how much of a substance can be removed from the blood by the kidneys per a unit of time.

54. Plasma creatinine concentration _____ when the GFR decreases, but it takes 7 to 10 days for the level

to stabilize, so this measure is best for monitoring _____ renal disease.

55. The BUN level _____ when the GFR decreases, but also varies with dehydration, protein intake, and

protein _____, which may make it unreliable for monitoring renal function.

FINISH THE DESCRIPTIONS

Finish these descriptions of physiologic processes by writing or drawing in the spaces provided.

56. **Micturition reflex:** As the bladder fills with urine, it begins to stretch. Mechanoreceptors in the bladder wall send neural sensory messages of stretch to the spinal cord. What happens next?

57. **Renal autoregulation:** With arterial blood pressures between 80 and 180 mm Hg, an increase of arterial blood pressure influences renal afferent arterioles in what way? Why is that important?

58. **Renin-angiotensin-aldosterone system:** Decreased blood flow through the renal artery stimulates the release of renin into the blood. What happens next? Describe the process until it has influenced renal function.

Chapter **29 Structure and Function of the Renal and Urologic Systems**

Write your response to each situation in the space provided.

59. Mr. Tyson, who is a plumber, says, "I understand that the ureters are tubes that carry urine from the kidney to the bladder. Gravity would move the urine down when a person is upright. But why does urine go through the ureters when a person is lying down?"

60. A nursing student says, "If 20% of the arterial blood that enters the kidneys is filtered into the renal tubules at the glomerulus, what happens to the other 80% that stays in the glomerulus after it leaves the efferent arterioles? Does it just leave the kidney by way of veins?"

61. A medical assistant in a refugee camp working with protein-malnourished people says, "I am surprised that even when our new refugees obviously are dehydrated, they still do not have the small quantities of dark yellow urine I would expect. They make larger amounts of lighter yellow urine. Why?"

62. "I am learning how the kidneys work," says Mrs. Boulpaep. "It says here that the glomeruli in the kidneys filter about 180 liters per day. I know we do not have that much fluid in our bodies! Is this number an error, or if it is true, why aren't we dead from urinating out our body fluids?"

63. "I wake up every night needing to urinate," says a retired nurse, age 78. "I know that age-related nocturia is normal, but I forget what basic changes in the kidney make that happen. Please explain."

30 Alterations of Renal and Urinary Tract Function

MATCH THE DEFINITIONS

Match each word on the right with its definition on the left.

_____ 1. Dilation of a ureter by accumulated urine

_____ 2. Enlargement of the renal pelvis and calyces by accumulated urine

_____ 3. Narrowing of the lumen of a urethra

_____ 4. Large urinary stone that has assumed the shape of the renal pelvis and calyces

A. Hydronephrosis

B. Staghorn calculus

C. Hydroureter

D. Urethral stricture

CIRCLE THE CORRECT WORDS

Circle the correct word from the choices provided to complete these sentences.

5. In addition to relieving pain, rapid removal of an upper urinary tract obstruction is important because the accumulating urine causes back pressure that (kills, hyperstimulates) renal cells.

6. When one kidney develops irreversible damage, the other kidney (makes additional nephrons, undergoes hypertrophy of existing glomeruli and tubules).

7. An alkaline urinary pH significantly increases the risk for (calcium phosphate, uric acid) stone formation, whereas acidic urine increases the risk for a (calcium phosphate, uric acid) stone.

8. The technical term for bladder dysfunction caused by neurologic disorders is (detrusor hyperreflexia, neurogenic bladder).

9. Cigarette smoking, arsenic in drinking water, and exposure to aniline dyes are risk factors for (renal, bladder) cancer, which is characterized by (painless, pain and) hematuria.

10. The most common route by which bacteria reach the bladder is (through the blood, retrograde up the urethra); the most common route by which bacteria reach the kidney is (through the blood, retrograde up a ureter).

11. The only manifestation of cystitis in an older adult may be the development of (confusion, headache).

12. Acute pyelonephritis primarily affects the (glomeruli, renal tubules) and is associated with sudden onset of fever, chills, and flank or groin (rash, pain).

13. The terms membranoproliferative glomerulonephritis and mesangial proliferative glomerulonephritis refer to the (clinical course, histologic appearance) of the condition.

14. Proteinuria and angiotensin II contribute to (reversible, irreversible) renal damage in (acute kidney injury, chronic kidney disease).

CATEGORIZE THE CAUSES

Write the type of acute kidney injury beside each cause. Choices: prerenal, intrarenal, postrenal.

_____ 15. Nephrotoxic antibiotics

_____ 16. Massive hemorrhage

_____ 17. Renal ischemia during surgery

_____ 18. Bilateral renal calculi

_____ 19. Untreated enlarged prostate

IDENTIFY THE EXAMPLES

Match the type of incontinence on the right with its example on the left.

_____ 20. A man was mildly confused, and his family brought him to adult day care during the week. He was incontinent there every day until a nurse suggested that they put a picture of a toilet on the bathroom door, and he became continent.

A. Urge incontinence

_____ 21. A woman has a bladder infection and is distressed to have episodes of sudden strong need to urinate that cause her to become incontinent.

B. Stress incontinence

_____ 22. A woman loses a small amount of urine involuntarily every time she sneezes.

C. Overflow incontinence

_____ 23. A man with a cauda equina involvement in multiple sclerosis became incontinent when his caregiver was late and was not available to assist with the morning catheterization.

D. Functional incontinence

DESCRIBE THE DIFFERENCES

Describe the difference between each pair of terms.

24. What is the difference between cystitis and pyelonephritis?

25. What is the difference between azotemia and uremia?

COMPLETE THE SENTENCES

Write one word in each blank to complete these sentences.

26. Urinary stones, also called _____, most commonly are composed of _____ salts but may have a different composition, depending on the individual's risk factors and the characteristics of the urine.

27. Obstructions to urine flow in the lower urinary tract include enlargement of the _____ in men and prolapse of the _____ _____ in women.

28. The most common renal cancers are renal cell _____.

29. Women who have chronic symptoms of cystitis with negative urine cultures may have _____ cystitis.

30. The primary cause of the damage in acute glomerulonephritis is the _____ system.

31. Two disease processes associated with chronic glomerulonephritis are lupus and _____.

32. The older term acute renal failure has been replaced with the term _____ _____ _____; the older term chronic renal failure has been replaced with the term _____ _____ _____.

33. Oliguria is a urine output of less than _____ mL per 24 hours.

MATCH THE CLINICAL MANIFESTATIONS

Match the disorder on the right with its classic signs and symptoms on the left.

_____ 34. No symptoms in early stages; hematuria, dull flank pain, weight loss, anemia in late stages

_____ 35. Sudden onset of hematuria, red blood cell casts, mild proteinuria, plus edema, hypertension, and oliguria if severe; may be asymptomatic

_____ 36. Severe colicky flank pain radiating to the groin, nausea and vomiting, some hematuria

_____ 37. Urgency, with or without urge incontinence, associated with frequency and nocturia, no bacteria in urine

_____ 38. Frequency, urgency, dysuria, suprapubic and low back pain, cloudy urine

_____ 39. Massive proteinuria, hypoproteinemia, hyperlipidemia, edema

_____ 40. Sudden onset of oliguria with elevated plasma BUN and plasma creatinine levels

A. Calculus lodged in ureter

B. Acute cystitis

C. Overactive bladder

D. Renal cancer

E. Acute kidney injury

F. Acute glomerulonephritis

G. Nephrotic syndrome

COMPLETE THE TABLE

Complete this table to figure out aspects of the uremic syndrome.

Normal Renal Function	Result of Impaired Function in the Uremic Syndrome
Excrete nitrogenous wastes	
Excrete potassium ions	
Excrete metabolic acids	
Excrete phosphate	
Activate vitamin D	
Secrete erythropoietin	
Excrete sodium and water	

Write your response to each situation in the space provided.

41. "I heard the medical student tell the doctor there are casts in my urine," says Mrs. Masterson, who has pyelonephritis. "What are casts?"

42. "I have a bladder infection," says Mrs. Barr, who is pregnant for the first time. "Why did my obstetrician tell me to call his office immediately if I get chills and fever?"

43. "Why am I so tired all the time?" says Mr. Rao, who has newly diagnosed end-stage chronic kidney disease. "Is that part of my kidney disease?"

44. "Why did the dialysis nurse tell me not to eat a lot of strawberries?" says Mr. Snyder, who has end-stage chronic kidney disease. "I love strawberry shortcake!"

45. "The nephrologist said my kidneys are damaged," says Mr. Lee, who has diabetes. "But I make so much urine that I get up three times in the night to urinate. She must be wrong."

46. "The doctor said I have hydronephrosis," says Mr. Boulet. "I thought I had a big kidney stone in my ureter. What is going on?"

47. "My patient has acute tubular necrosis," says a nurse. "I took care of him for over 2 weeks, and he had oliguria. After my days off, I come back and find that he has mild polyuria. I am really worried at this change, but no one else is. What is going on?"

48. "Why do people who have nephrotic syndrome have so much protein in their urine?" asks a nurse who is new to the renal unit. "Do they have big holes in their glomeruli?"

49. A woman approaches a physician assistant at a community blood pressure screening. "I need to know what stress incontinence is," she says. "Tell me first and then I'll explain why I ask."

50. Mrs. Hixon, who has type 2 diabetes, has newly diagnosed end-stage chronic kidney disease. A nurse who enters Mrs. Hixon's hospital room sees a big box of raisins on the bedside table. Mrs. Hixon smiles and says, "My physician said I am anemic, so I asked my husband to bring me some raisins. That's what I ate years ago when I got anemic from menstruating so heavily. That cured it!" How should the nurse respond?

51. A newly employed nurse at a neurologic injury rehabilitation facility says, "Please help me make sense of the bladder dysfunctions after neurologic injury. Some of our patients have underactive bladders, and others have overactive bladders. What makes the difference?"

Chapter **30** **Alterations of Renal and Urinary Tract Function**

31 Alterations of Renal and Urinary Tract Function in Children

MATCH THE DEFINITIONS

Match each word on the right with its definition on the left.

_____ 1. Congenital condition in which the urethral meatus is located on the ventral surface of the penis

_____ 2. Ventral bend of the penis

_____ 3. Absence of one or both kidneys

_____ 4. Small kidney with decreased number of nephrons

A. Chordee

B. Hypoplastic kidney

C. Renal agenesis

D. Hypospadias

CIRCLE THE CORRECT WORDS

Circle the correct word from the choices provided to complete these sentences.

5. Bladder infection, also known as (cystitis, bladderitis), causes detrusor muscle hyperactivity that (increases, decreases) bladder capacity.

6. Childhood urinary tract infections are most common in (girls, boys) aged 7 to 11.

7. Differentiating between bladder and kidney infection in children is (easy, difficult); one indicator is that UTI in a previously toilet-trained child may cause (enuresis, hyperactivity).

8. Most children acquire bladder control before (2, 5) years of age.

9. Primary nephrotic syndrome also is known as (functional, idiopathic) nephrotic syndrome and occurs in the (presence, absence) of preexisting systemic disease.

10. Presence of a urethral valve obstructs the (bladder outlet, kidney outflow).

EXPLAIN THE PICTURES

Examine the pictures and answer the questions about them.

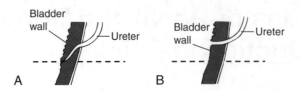

11. These pictures show the insertion of a ureter into the bladder wall. What is the difference in the angle at which the ureter travels through the bladder wall in picture B compared with picture A?

12. Which picture shows the normal anatomy? _____

13. The abnormal insertion angle of the ureter is associated with what condition?

_____

14. What happens when the bladder muscle contracts in this condition?

15. How does this condition predispose to cystitis and pyelonephritis?

DESCRIBE THE DIFFERENCES

Describe the difference between each pair of terms.

16. What is the difference between hypospadias and epispadias in males?

17. What is the difference between a hypoplastic kidney and a dysplastic kidney?

18. What is the difference between primary incontinence and secondary incontinence?

19. What is the difference between chordee and penile torsion?

COMPLETE THE SENTENCES

Write one word in each blank to complete these sentences.

20. When kidneys fuse in the midline as they ascend during development, the U-shaped kidney is called a _____ kidney.

21. Failure of the abdominal muscles and anterior bladder to fuse in the midline with subsequent exposure of the posterior bladder mucosa is called _____ of the bladder.

22. Blockage of the tapered point where the renal pelvis transitions into the ureter is called _____ _____ obstruction and causes _____ in neonates.

23. Another name for Wilms tumor is _____, a tumor of the _____ that usually presents as an enlarging, firm, nontender smooth mass on one side of the _____.

24. Nephrotic syndrome is characterized by proteinuria, _____, hyperlipidemia, and _____ that often is _____ in the morning and more evident in the abdomen and lower extremities later in the day.

TEACH PEOPLE ABOUT PATHOPHYSIOLOGY

Write your response to each situation in the space provided.

25. "Why is Keely's urine foamy?" says Keely's mother. "Is that part of her nephrotic syndrome?"

26. "My mother had polycystic kidney disease too," says Jason Frei, age 15, who has just learned that he has the condition. "I have always wondered what polycystic means."

27. Mrs. Garrow's infant died a few hours after birth because of Potter's syndrome. "The doctor said my baby had no kidneys and that is why his lungs went bad," she says. "Please explain that."

Read the case scenario and answer the questions to explore your understanding of glomerulonephritis.

Shane Nye, age 9, had a severe sore throat that was diagnosed as "strep throat" at a clinic visit. His mother was given a prescription for an antibiotic, which she did not fill because she received notice that her electricity would be cut off if she did not pay her overdue bill immediately. After paying her electric bill, she had no money left. Ten days later, Shane's urine became smoky brown, and he did not feel well. His ankles were slightly swollen, so his mother took him to a free clinic. Shane's diagnosis is acute poststreptococcal glomerulonephritis.

28. "Did the strep infect Shane's kidneys?" asks Mrs. Nye. "I did not have any money for that antibiotic." What should the clinic nurse respond?

29. Why is Shane's urine smoky brown?

30. Why did Shane's ankles swell?

31. What role do antigen-antibody complexes play in the pathophysiology of acute poststreptococcal glomerulonephritis?

32. Other types of glomerulonephritis also cause hematuria in children. How do the clinical manifestations of Henoch-Schönlein purpura nephritis differ from this case scenario?

32 Structure and Function of the Reproductive Systems

MATCH THE DEFINITIONS

Match each word on the right with its definition on the left.

_____ 1. Onset of sexual maturation

_____ 2. Maturation of the ovaries or testes

_____ 3. Onset of menstruation

_____ 4. Onset of breast development

_____ 5. Increased production of adrenal androgens before puberty

A. Thelarche

B. Puberty

C. Gonadarche

D. Adrenarche

E. Menarche

CIRCLE THE CORRECT WORDS

Circle the correct word from the choices provided to complete these sentences.

6. Production of ova (occurs only during fetal life, begins at puberty); production of sperm (occurs only during fetal life; begins at puberty).

7. Menopause is defined as cessation of menstrual flow for (3 months if not pregnant, 1 year).

8. A vaginal pH that is (low, high) protects against infection.

9. The most important estrogen is E2, also known as (estriol, estradiol).

10. Ovulation is triggered by a surge of (LH and FSH, ACTH) from the (posterior, anterior) pituitary, controlled by (GnRH, CRF) from the hypothalamus.

11. Maintaining pregnancy is an important function of the hormone (estrogen, progesterone).

12. The characteristic hormone profile of menopause is (low, high) estrogen and progesterone levels and (low, high) FSH and LH levels.

ORDER THE STEPS

Sequence the events that occur during spermatogenesis.

13. Write the letters here in the correct order of the steps: _____
    A. Sperm cells migrate to the epididymis.
    B. Spermatogonia divide by mitosis.
    C. Spermatids attach to Sertoli cells and mature into sperm cells.
    D. Primary and secondary spermatocytes divide by meiosis.
    E. Sperm become motile when activated by biochemicals in semen.

EXPLAIN THE PICTURES

Examine the pictures and answer the questions about them.

UNDIFFERENTIATED

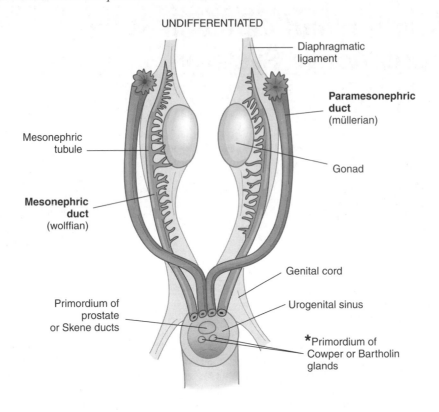

This picture shows embryonic reproductive structures that have not yet differentiated.

14. Expression of a gene on the _____ chromosome creates TDF, a determining factor that stimulates the gonads to develop into _____.

15. In the absence of a Y chromosome, expression of other genes causes the gonads to develop into _____ and triggers regression of which of type of duct in the picture? _____

16. What happens to the remaining ducts in the presence of estrogen and absence of appreciable amounts of testosterone?

17. The primordium marked with an asterisk (*) in the picture will develop into Cowper glands in a _____ and Bartholin glands in a _____.

18. What analogous function do those glands serve in sexually mature adults? ·

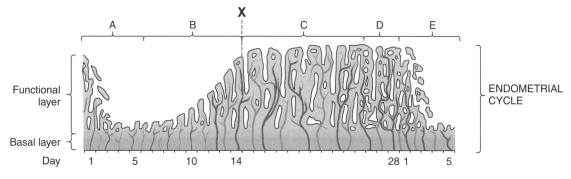

(Adapted from Lowdermilk DL, et al: *Maternity nursing & women's health care,* ed 10, St Louis, 2012, Mosby.)

19. The phases of the endometrial cycle are labeled with letters. What words do the letters indicate?

    A = _____; B = _____; C = _____; D =_____; E = _____

20. Which phase of the endometrial cycle occurs during the luteal phase of the ovarian cycle? _____

21. What hormone produced by the ovary is in greatest supply during the luteal phase of the ovarian cycle?

    _____

22. What hormone produced by the ovary is responsible for the endometrial events in phase B? _____

23. What occurs at the point marked X in the picture? _____

DESCRIBE THE DIFFERENCES

Describe the difference between each pair of terms.

24. What is the difference between puberty and adolescence?

25. What is the difference between menarche and menopause?

COMPLETE THE SENTENCES

Write one word in each blank to complete these sentences.

26. A gamete has _____ chromosomes.

27. The female structure analogous to the male penis is the _____.

28. The functional layer of the _____ sloughs off during menstruation, but the _____ layer remains and regenerates the functional layer.

Chapter **32** **Structure and Function of the Reproductive Systems**

29. The portion of the uterus located above the insertion of the fallopian tubes is called the _____.

30. After the release of an ovum, an ovarian follicle becomes the _____ _____.

31. In females, LH stimulates theca cells in the primary follicle to produce _____; in males, LH stimulates Leydig cells to produce _____.

32. Although menstrual (ovarian) cycles can vary in length, the _____ phase is relatively fixed at 14 days.

33. The usual site of fertilization of an ovum is in the _____ _____.

TEACH PEOPLE ABOUT PHYSIOLOGY

Write your response to each situation in the space provided.

34. Mrs. Yarnold, age 74, says, "I never had a vaginal infection when I was young, but now that I am older, I have had two. I still keep good hygiene. Why would I get infections now?"

35. Ms. Francisco, age 34, is looking at a diagram of the female reproductive system. "Look at those lovely fringes on the ends of the fallopian tubes," she says. "Do they have any useful purpose?"

36. Ms. Lendler, age 36, says, "My nurse practitioner told me to wait to schedule my mammogram until right after my menstrual period. Is there a good reason for that timing?"

37. Mr. Martinelli says, "My wife and I want to have a baby. Her nurse practitioner told my wife to ask me to stay out of the hot tub until my wife gets pregnant. Why?"

33 Alterations of the Female Reproductive System

MATCH THE DEFINITIONS

Match each word on the right with its definition on the left.

_____ 1. Development of the breasts in girls	A. Hirsutism
_____ 2. The process of sexual maturation	B. Cystocele
_____ 3. Menstrual cycles longer than 6 to 7 weeks	C. Enterocele
_____ 4. Abnormal hairiness	D. Puberty
_____ 5. Heavy or irregular bleeding in the absence of organic disease	E. Thelarche
_____ 6. Bulging of the rectum and posterior vaginal wall into the vaginal canal	F. Leiomyoma
_____ 7. Descent of a portion of the posterior bladder wall and trigone into the vaginal canal	G. Dysfunctional uterine bleeding
_____ 8. Herniation of the rectouterine pouch into the septum between the rectum and posterior vaginal wall	H. Oligomenorrhea
_____ 9. Benign smooth muscle tumor in the uterine muscle	I. Rectocele

CIRCLE THE CORRECT WORDS

Circle the correct word from the choices provided to complete these sentences.

10. Premenstrual syndrome and premenstrual dysphoric disorder occur during the (luteal, follicular) phase of the menstrual cycle.

11. During the reproductive years, the (acid, alkaline) pH of the vagina protects against infection.

12. Vulvodynia is (chronic pain of, cyst formation in) the vulva; a Bartholin cyst occurs in the (duct, gland body) of the Bartholin gland.

13. Risk factors for pelvic organ prolapse include (very low body weight, obesity), familial tendency, childbirth, and (abdominal, pelvic) surgery or trauma.

14. Endometrial polyps are often related to (estrogen, progesterone) stimulation and are a common cause of (scanty, excessive) menstrual bleeding.

15. HPV-associated carcinoma in situ is most likely to develop where the (squamous, columnar) epithelium of the cervical lining meets the (squamous, columnar) epithelium of the outer cervix and vagina.

16. Most cervical cancers are (symptomatic; asymptomatic); the major symptom of invasive vaginal cancer is vaginal (dryness, bleeding).

17. The major risk factor for endometrial cancer is prolonged exposure to (estrogen, progesterone) without the presence of (estrogen, progesterone).

18. Nonproliferative breast lesions generally (are, are not) associated with an increased risk for breast cancer; an example of a nonproliferative breast lesion is (ductal hyperplasia, fibrocystic disease).

19. Involuntary muscle spasm that prevents penetration during sexual intercourse is termed (dyspareunia, vaginismus).

EXPLAIN THE PICTURES

Examine the pictures and answer the questions about them.

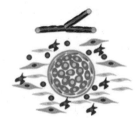 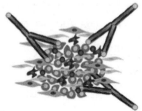

A Ductal carcinoma in situ   B Advanced breast cancer

20. What is the difference between the disorders in Figure A and Figure B with regard to the basement membrane?

21. Will the DCIS in Figure A invariably progress to the cancer in Figure B? _____

22. Which figure shows a lesion that might be detected clinically as a lump? _____

23. Would that lump typically be painful or painless? _____

24. Is it likely that the cells in the cancer in Figure B are homogeneous? Explain your answer.

CATEGORIZE THE RISK FACTORS

Write the classification beside each risk factor for breast cancer. Choices: reproductive, hormonal, familial, environmental.

_____ 25. BRCA2 mutation

_____ 26. High alcohol consumption

_____ 27. Nulliparity

_____ 28. Cigarette smoking

_____ 29. Late menopause

_____ 30. Physical inactivity

_____ 31. Excess radiation to breasts

_____ 32. Menopausal hormone therapy

_____ 33. Breast cancer in first-degree relative

DESCRIBE THE DIFFERENCES

Describe the difference between each pair of terms.

34. What is the difference between primary and secondary dysmenorrhea?

35. What is the difference between primary and secondary amenorrhea?

36. What is the difference between menorrhagia and metrorrhagia?

37. What is the difference between vaginitis and vaginosis?

38. What is the difference between endometriosis and adenomyosis?

COMPLETE THE SENTENCES

Write one word in each blank to complete these sentences.

39. Puberty is considered delayed if there are no clinical signs of puberty by age _____ in girls.

40. Precocious puberty is sexual maturation before age _____ in black girls or age _____ in white girls and before age _____ in boys.

41. The most common cause of secondary dysmenorrhea is _____.

42. Primary amenorrhea can arise from failure of the _____ to synthesize GnRH, failure of the _____ pituitary to synthesize _____ and LH, failure of the ovaries to secrete _____, or anatomic defects of the uterus or vagina.

43. Inflammation of the fallopian tubes is termed _____ and is categorized as _____ _____ disease.

44. Ovarian cysts that may contain mature tissue such as muscle fibers or bone are called _____ cysts.

45. Oncogenic strains 16 and 18 of _____ _____ virus cause _____ cancer.

46. Inappropriate lactation is called _____; a common cause is excessive production of the hormone

_____, often from a tumor in the anterior _____.

TEACH PEOPLE ABOUT PATHOPHYSIOLOGY

Write your response to each situation in the space provided.

47. "Oh no! My cousin couldn't get pregnant and have a baby after she had gonorrhea!" says Ms. Sokol when she learns that she has gonorrhea. After Ms. Sokol leaves, a student nurse says, "Gonorrhea is treatable with antibiotics. How could gonorrhea interfere with pregnancy?"

48. Mrs. Strider had a dense area on a mammogram and was worried that she had breast cancer. A biopsy of the area showed that she has fibrocystic breast disease. "I am so glad that the biopsy showed no cancer!" says Mrs. Strider. "What is fibrocystic breast disease?"

49. Ms. Chavez says, "Every time I have to take antibiotics for a bladder infection, I get a vaginal yeast infection! Why is that?"

50. A physician assistant says, "I understand the normal ovarian cycle and the formation of the dominant follicle during the ovarian cycle. But what goes wrong when a woman develops an ovarian follicular cyst?"

51. Mrs. Jacobs has endometriosis. She asks, "Why does it hurt the most when I am menstruating?"

52. Mrs. Kepler had vaginal bleeding 3 years after menopause and was diagnosed with uterine cancer. She says, "I guess I am not totally unlucky; I hear the death rate is higher with ovarian cancer. Please tell me why that death rate is higher."

Read the clinical scenarios and answer the questions to explore your understanding of pelvic inflammatory disease and polycystic ovary syndrome.

Jodie Nickelson, a 20-year-old college student, visits the student health center because she has pelvic pain. She reports the recent development of pain with intercourse and with defecation, dyspareunia, and dysmenorrhea. Her pelvic pain increases greatly if she jumps or tries to walk briskly. Jodie states that she is sexually active but is on oral contraceptives and is currently experiencing her normal menstrual period.

Physical Examination

■ Temperature 100.0° F (37.8° C); HR, BP, and respirations within normal limits

■ Tenderness on cervical movement during pelvic examination

Jodie's diagnosis is pelvic inflammatory disease (PID).

53. Why did the nurse practitioner measure Jodie's temperature?

54. What organs are commonly involved in PID?

55. What is the technical term for pain with sexual intercourse? _____

56. What is the technical term for pain with defecation? _____

57. Why does pain occur with sexual intercourse and defecation in PID?

58. During the pelvic examination, Jodie experienced pain with cervical movement. Why is this an expected finding in her situation?

59. Jodie was treated successfully with antibiotics. What potential complications of PID might Jodie experience in the future?

Marge Orrin, age 28, visited a woman's health care nurse practitioner because she was unable to become pregnant after trying for a year.

History

- Menses have been irregular since menarche

- Typically has five menses per year, with heavy bleeding that is heavier in the past year

- Last menstrual period 3 weeks ago

- Weight gain of 40 pounds in past 18 months

- Mother had chin hair that she shaved regularly

Physical Examination

- BP 144/90; other vital signs within normal limits

- Weight 251 pounds, BMI 35.4

- Dark hair on chin and chest

- Moderate acne on back

- No acanthosis nigricans

- Obese abdomen, no tenderness

- Normal external genitalia, no clitoromegaly

Laboratory Tests

- TSH and prolactin normal

- Testosterone elevated

- LDL elevated

- Pelvic ultrasound showed polycystic ovaries

Mrs. Orrin's diagnoses were polycystic ovary syndrome (PCOS) and hypertension.

60. What clinical effects of excess androgens did Mrs. Orrin have?

61. What are the typical blood levels of androgens in PCOS? Circle the correct answer.

Increased   Normal   Decreased

62. What are the typical blood levels of estrogens in PCOS? Circle the correct answer.

    Increased   Normal   Decreased

63. What is the significance of Mrs. Orrin's BMI in the context of PCOS?

64. How do elevated androgens and insulin contribute to the abnormal ovarian follicle development in PCOS?

Chapter **33 Alterations of the Female Reproductive System**

34 Alterations of the Male Reproductive System

MATCH THE DEFINITIONS

Match each word on the right with its definition on the left.

_____ 1. Visible enlargement of breast tissue in a male

_____ 2. Foreskin of the penis

_____ 3. Narrowing of the urethra due to scarring

_____ 4. Prolonged painful penile erection

_____ 5. Inflammation of the glans penis

_____ 6. Fibrosis of the corpora cavernosa that causes penile curvature during erection

_____ 7. Undescended testicle (or both testes)

_____ 8. Inflammation of the testes

_____ 9. Inflammation of the foreskin

_____ 10. Cyst in the epididymis

_____ 11. Abnormally dilated vein within the spermatic cord

A. Peyronie disease

B. Cryptorchidism

C. Balanitis

D. Orchitis

E. Spermatocele

F. Posthitis

G. Varicocele

H. Urethral stricture

I. Prepuce

J. Priapism

K. Gynecomastia

CIRCLE THE CORRECT WORDS

Circle the correct word from the choices provided to complete these sentences.

12. Most breast cancers in men are (estrogen, androgen) positive.

13. Any factor that causes testicular temperature to (fall, rise) can impair sperm production.

14. Most penile cancer is (squamous cell carcinoma, adenocarcinoma), whereas most prostate cancer is (squamous cell carcinoma, adenocarcinoma).

15. The most common infectious cause of orchitis in postpubertal males is (gonorrhea, mumps).

16. Testicular torsion requires immediate treatment to prevent (ischemia and necrosis, epididymitis and sterility).

17. Benign prostatic hyperplasia (BPH) begins in the (inner layers, periphery) of the prostate; most prostate cancer begins in the (inner layers, periphery) of the prostate.

18. In acute bacterial prostatitis, bacteria reach the prostate (through the blood, by ascending the urinary tract); the clinical manifestations are similar to those of (pyelonephritis, prostate cancer).

19. Arterial diseases can cause sexual dysfunction by interfering with (erection, ejaculation).

DESCRIBE THE DIFFERENCES

Describe the difference between each pair of terms.

20. What is the difference between phimosis and paraphimosis?

21. What is the difference between delayed puberty and precocious puberty in boys?

22. What is the difference between a varicocele and a hydrocele?

COMPLETE THE SENTENCES

Write one word in each blank to complete these sentences.

23. The most common type of testicular cancer is _____, the least aggressive type.

24. Urine reflux into the epididymis causes _____ _____.

25. The prostate and other tissues use the enzyme aromatase to convert androgens to _____.

26. Sexual dysfunction is impairment of any of these three processes (listed in the order that they normally occur): _____, _____, _____.

27. Gynecomastia often involves imbalance of the _____ ratio.

TEACH PEOPLE ABOUT PATHOPHYSIOLOGY

Write your response to each situation in the space provided.

28. Mr. Marcum has been diagnosed with BPH. He says, "Tell me why it takes so long for me to empty my bladder."

29. Mr. Hoover says, "My 90-year-old uncle has prostate cancer, but the doctor said to watch and wait rather than do surgery! Why? Isn't cancer fatal? He is healthy otherwise."

30. Mr. Ortega had burning on urination and went to see a nurse practitioner. He was diagnosed with nongonococcal urethritis. He says, "I know what urethritis means, but what about nongonococcal? Do I have gonorrhea?"

31. Mr. Singh went to a clinic because he has a scrotal mass. Afterward, he says, "That doctor says I have a hydrocele and not to worry, but I am not sure he knows what he is doing! Why did he put a flashlight in back of my scrotum and look at it?"

32. Mr. Watson, age 33, noticed that that his right testicle was enlarged. It did not hurt. His physician palpated Mr. Watson's testes, discovered a firm mass in the enlarged testicle, and made an appointment for Mr. Watson to have an ultrasound examination. Mr. Watson says, "I know my doctor is concerned that I might have testicular cancer, but why did he ask me if I had undescended testicles when I was an infant? And why did he feel my groin after he found the mass in my testicle?"

35 Structure and Function of the Digestive System

MATCH THE DEFINITIONS

Match each word on the right with its definition on the left.

_____	1. Waves of sequential relaxations and contractions of the gastrointestinal muscles	A. Segmentation
_____	2. The functional units of the small intestine	B. Chyme
_____	3. An iron-binding protein	C. Peristalsis
_____	4. Localized rhythmic contractions of intestinal circular smooth muscles that are not peristalsis	D. Villi
_____	5. Partially digested food in the stomach and intestine	E. Transferrin

MATCH THE CELLS

Match the cell on the right with its function on the left.

_____	6. Metabolize nutrients, detoxify chemicals, secrete bile, synthesize albumin and clotting factors, and other functions	A. Kupffer cells
_____	7. Remove bacteria and foreign particles from blood in the hepatic sinusoids	B. Pancreatic acinar cells
_____	8. Secrete digestive proenzymes	C. Pancreatic ductal epithelium
_____	9. Secrete bicarbonate-rich fluid	D. Hepatocytes
_____	10. Secrete gastrin	E. Enterochromaffin-like cells
_____	11. Secrete hydrochloric acid and intrinsic factor	F. Chief cells
_____	12. Secrete gastric histamine	G. G cells
_____	13. Secrete gastric somatostatin	H. Parietal cells
_____	14. Secrete pepsinogen	I. D cells

CIRCLE THE CORRECT WORDS

Circle the correct word from the choices provided to complete these sentences.

15. Gastrin and motilin (stimulate, delay) gastric emptying; secretin and cholecystokinin (stimulate, delay) gastric emptying.

16. The (gallbladder, liver) produces bile, which is slightly (acidic, alkaline).

17. The composition of saliva depends on the rate of (eating, its secretion).

18. Saliva contains (lymphocytes, immunoglobulin A), which can help prevent infection.

19. Stretching the esophagus or intestine by a bolus of food causes (peristalsis, relaxation).

20. Fatty foods (stimulate, delay) gastric emptying; hypertonic gastric contents (stimulate, delay) gastric emptying.

21. The intestinal brush border is the collection of (villi, microvilli).

22. Most of the water that enters the gastrointestinal tract each day is absorbed in the (small, large) intestine; sugars are absorbed primarily in the (initial, terminal) portions of the (small, large) intestine.

23. The intestinal tract is (sterile, partially colonized) at birth and becomes totally colonized within 3 to 4 (days, weeks).

24. A choleretic agent is a substance that stimulates the (pancreas, liver) to secrete (bile, glucagon).

25. Pancreatic proteases are secreted in (active, inactive) form; pancreatic amylases are secreted in (active, inactive) form; pancreatic lipases are secreted in (active, inactive) form.

26. As age increases, gastrointestinal motility tends to (increase, decrease), and liver blood flow and enzyme activity tend to (increase, decrease).

CATEGORIZE THE STIMULI

Write the action of each stimulus on secretion of gastric acid. Choices: increase, decrease.

_____ 27. Histamine

_____ 28. Cholecystokinin

_____ 29. Gastrin

_____ 30. Increased vagal stimulation

_____ 31. Increased sympathetic stimulation

_____ 32. Caffeine

ORDER THE STEPS

Ending with the formation of bile, sequence the events that occur with the heme when an aged red blood cell is destroyed in the spleen.

33. Write the letters here in the correct order of the steps: _____
    A. Unconjugated bilirubin binds to albumin and circulates to the liver.
    B. Aged erythrocyte is destroyed by macrophages in the spleen.
    C. Unconjugated bilirubin enters the liver sinusoids and then the hepatocytes.
    D. Macrophages separate heme from the remainder of the hemoglobin, converting it to biliverdin.
    E. Hepatocytes conjugate bilirubin and secrete it into bile.
    F. Macrophages convert biliverdin to unconjugated bilirubin.

EXPLAIN THE PICTURE

Examine the picture and answer the questions about it.

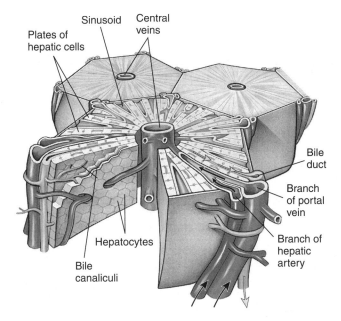

34. This drawing shows internal architecture of what organ? _____

35. What term is used to describe the structure that surrounds the central veins? (Hint: This drawing shows three of these structures.)

_____

36. What structures lie between sheets of hepatocytes?

_____

37. What is the source of the blood that enters the sinusoids?

_____

38. The sinusoids drain into what blood vessels?

_____

39. Why is it important that the sinusoids are lined with highly permeable endothelium?

_____

40. The hepatocytes secrete bile into what structures?

_____

DESCRIBE THE DIFFERENCES

Describe the difference between each pair of terms.

41. What is the difference between the esophageal wall muscles in the upper part and the lower part of the esophagus?

42. What is the difference between the visceral and parietal peritoneum?

43. What is the difference between the gastric antrum and the gastric fundus?

Chapter **35 Structure and Function of the Digestive System**

44. What is the difference between a micelle and a chylomicron?

MATCH THE ENZYMES

Match the enzyme on the right with its description on the left.

_____ 45. Pancreatic enzyme that digests proteins

_____ 46. Gastric enzyme that digests proteins

_____ 47. Salivary enzyme that digests carbohydrates

_____ 48. Pancreatic enzyme that digests carbohydrates

_____ 49. Intestinal enzyme that digests disaccharides

_____ 50. Pancreatic enzyme that digests fats

A. Lipase

B. Amylase

C. Maltase

D. Ptyalin

E. Trypsin

F. Pepsin

COMPLETE THE SENTENCES

Write one word in each blank to complete these sentences.

51. Branches of the _____ artery provide most of the blood to the stomach; the _____ _____ artery provides most of the blood to the small intestine.

52. The three segments of the small intestine, in order, are _____, _____, and _____.

53. The center of every villus has a lymphatic capillary that is known as a _____ that is important for absorption of _____ molecules.

54. In the intestines, _____ occurs in the crypts, and _____ occurs at the tops of the villi.

55. The _____ sphincter marks the junction between the stomach and the duodenum; the sphincter of _____ marks the junction between the bile duct and the duodenum.

56. The _____ valve marks the junction between the terminal ileum and the large intestine; this valve normally is _____ to prevent retrograde flow of intestinal contents.

57. The four parts of the colon, in order, are the ascending colon, _____ colon, _____ colon, and _____ colon.

58. The internal anal sphincter contains _____ muscle; the external anal sphincter contains _____ muscle.

59. The _____ ligament is the remnant of the umbilical vein; the _____ ligament separates the right and left lobes of the liver and attaches it to the anterior _____ wall.

60. Hepatocytes synthesize the primary bile acids from _____; the body recycles bile acids through the process of _____ circulation.

61. The hormone _____ activates trypsinogen in the duodenum.

62. The layers of the stomach and intestinal walls, in order beginning at the lumen, are the mucosa, _____, _____, and serosa.

63. The _____ nervous system lies within the gastrointestinal tract and consists of neurons of the submucosal plexus, the _____ plexus, and the subserosal plexus.

TEACH PEOPLE ABOUT PHYSIOLOGY

Write your response to each situation in the space provided.

64. Mr. Hazzard learned that ibuprofen, his favorite analgesic, decreases the mucus in the stomach. He says, "Why should I care about mucus in the stomach?"

65. Frank, age 17, is learning about digestion. He says, "Why doesn't the pepsin from the stomach digest the protein in the walls of the small intestine?"

66. Mrs. Easton, a retired chemist, has a prescription for iron supplements because she has iron deficiency anemia. She says, "Why did the physician assistant tell me to take vitamin C when I take my iron pill?"

67. Mrs. Hamilton's son has appendicitis. "I know the appendix is in the belly," she says, "but where is it attached?

68. Mrs. Lee says, "My nurse practitioner told me to go sit on the toilet right after eating, to take advantage of the gastrocolic reflex. What is that?"

69. Mr. Thomas, a butcher, says, "Every time I see a gallbladder, I wonder what good is bile. Can you tell me?"

36 Alterations of Digestive Function

MATCH THE DEFINITIONS

Match each word on the right with its definition on the left.

_____ 1. Difficulty swallowing

_____ 2. Accumulation of fluid in the peritoneal cavity

_____ 3. Loss of appetite

_____ 4. Vomiting of blood

_____ 5. Dark, tarry stools

_____ 6. Frank bleeding from the rectum

_____ 7. Formation of gallstones

_____ 8. Physical wasting with weight loss, muscle atrophy, fatigue, and weakness

_____ 9. The muscular event of vomiting without the expulsion of vomitus

_____ 10. Distended, tortuous, collateral veins

A. Melena

B. Anorexia

C. Cholelithiasis

D. Dysphagia

E. Retching

F. Ascites

G. Cachexia

H. Hematochezia

I. Varices

J. Hematemesis

CIRCLE THE CORRECT WORDS

Circle the correct word from the choices provided to complete these sentences.

11. People who have GERD have (increased, decreased) resting tone of the (upper, lower) esophageal sphincter; the symptoms include heartburn and chronic (constipation, cough).

12. The most common type of hiatal hernia is (paraesophageal, sliding); this type (is, is not) associated with gastro-esophageal reflux.

13. Acute obstruction high in the small intestine causes (vomiting, constipation) first; acute obstruction low in the small intestine causes (vomiting, constipation) first.

14. With acute mesenteric arterial insufficiency, the damaged intestinal mucosa cannot produce enough mucus to protect itself from (acid, digestive enzymes); bacteria invade the (healthy, necrotic) intestinal wall, eventually causing (peritonitis, malabsorption).

15. Neurons in the (hypothalamus, cerebral cortex) play a major role in regulating appetite, food intake, and energy metabolism; hormones that circulate in the blood serve as (central, peripheral) signals to this area when their concentrations increase or decrease in relation to (body fat mass, liver function).

16. (Peripheral, Visceral) obesity is associated with a greater risk for metabolic syndrome, type 2 diabetes, and cardiovascular complications; resistance to (adiponectin, leptin) and decreased production of (adiponectin, leptin) contribute to the insulin resistance of obesity.

17. Cirrhosis and hepatitis can cause (posthepatic, intrahepatic) portal hypertension; severe right-sided heart failure can cause (posthepatic, intrahepatic) portal hypertension.

18. The most accepted theory of ascites formation involves the combination of portal (vasodilation, hypertension) and splanchnic arterial (vasodilation, hypertension); ascites can be complicated by (bacterial, viral) peritonitis.

19. The (blue, yellow) color of jaundice usually appears first in the (skin, sclera of the eye).

CATEGORIZE THE CLINICAL MANIFESTATIONS

Write the major cause beside each clinical manifestation of cirrhosis. Choices: portal hypertension, hepatocyte dysfunction.

_____ 20. Esophageal varices

_____ 21. Jaundice

_____ 22. Hepatic encephalopathy

_____ 23. Hemorrhoids

_____ 24. Splenomegaly

_____ 25. Caput medusae

_____ 26. Hypoalbuminemia

ORDER THE STEPS

Sequence the events that occur with an acute obstruction of the small intestine.

27. Write the letters here in the correct order of the steps: _____
    A. Decreased venous flow contributes to decreased arterial flow in the intestinal wall.
    B. Fluid and gas accumulate proximal to the obstruction, causing distention.
    C. Increased capillary permeability facilitates bacterial and fluid movement into the peritoneal cavity.
    D. The intestinal lumen becomes obstructed acutely.
    E. Edema and ischemia of the intestinal wall occur.
    F. Prolonged increase of tension in the intestinal wall collapses veins in the wall.
    G. Hypovolemia and peritonitis are likely.

CHARACTERIZE THE TYPES OF HEPATITIS

Characterize the types of hepatitis by completing this table.

Characteristic	Hepatitis A Infection	Hepatitis B Infection	Hepatitis C Infection	Hepatitis D Infection	Hepatitis E Infection
Route of transmission					
Acute or chronic?					
Carrier state					

DESCRIBE THE DIFFERENCES

Describe the difference between each pair of terms.

28. What is the difference between GERD and NERD?

29. What is the difference between type A and type B chronic gastritis?

30. What is the difference between maldigestion and malabsorption?

31. What is the difference between orexigenic neurons and anorexigenic neurons?

32. What is the difference between the metabolic pathways in short-term and long-term starvation?

33. What is the difference between alcoholic cirrhosis and biliary cirrhosis?

Chapter **36** **Alterations of Digestive Function**

MATCH THE DISORDERS

Match the disorder on the right with its description on the left.

_____ 34. Absence of an enzyme causes bloating, crampy pain, diarrhea, and flatulence after ingesting milk

_____ 35. A gastrointestinal disorder with unclear pathophysiology that is characterized by recurrent abdominal pain and altered bowel habits

_____ 36. Rapid gastric emptying of hypertonic chyme after bariatric surgery causes hypotension, pallor, cramping, nausea, and diarrhea

_____ 37. Asymptomatic presence of saclike outpouchings that are continuous with the GI tract lumen

_____ 38. Gastrin-secreting tumor causes gastric and duodenal ulcers, gastroesophageal reflux with abdominal pain, and diarrhea

_____ 39. Rapid provision of nutrients after starvation causes severe hypophosphatemia and other electrolyte imbalances that may be fatal

_____ 40. Inflammation of saclike outpouchings that are continuous with the GI tract lumen

_____ 41. Increased bilirubin, predominantly conjugated, in the blood caused by obstruction of the common bile duct

_____ 42. Increased bilirubin, both conjugated and unconjugated, in the blood caused by failure of liver cells to conjugate bilirubin and of bilirubin to pass from liver to intestine

_____ 43. Necrosis of liver cells without preexisting liver disease or cirrhosis, often because of acetaminophen overdose

A. Zollinger-Ellison syndrome

B. Lactase deficiency

C. Posthepatic jaundice

D. Dumping syndrome

E. Diverticulitis

F. Diverticulosis

G. Irritable bowel syndrome

H. Acute liver failure

I. Refeeding syndrome

J. Hepatocellular jaundice

COMPLETE THE SENTENCES

Write one word in each blank to complete these sentences.

44. Functional dysphagia caused by loss of esophageal innervation is called _____.

45. Protrusion of the upper part of the stomach through the diaphragm and into the thorax is called _____ _____.

46. People who have acute obstruction high in the small intestine are at risk for metabolic _____, but those with acute obstruction low in the small intestine are at risk for metabolic _____.

47. Acute gastritis often heals within a few _____, especially when injurious agents such as NSAIDs and alcohol are stopped.

48. Gastric ulcers and duodenal ulcers both are called _____ ulcers; risk factors include *H.* _____ and use of NSAIDs.

49. Although pancreatic insufficiency causes poor digestion of all nutrients, maldigestion of _____ because of lack of _____ is the chief problem.

50. Diverticula involve herniation of the _____ through the muscle layers; the most common location where diverticula develop is the _____.

51. Pain from appendicitis typically moves from the epigastric or _____ region to the _____ _____ quadrant.

52. Obesity is defined as a body mass index that exceeds _____ kg/m^2 and generally develops when caloric intake _____ caloric expenditure in genetically susceptible individuals.

53. Cytokines and hormones secreted by adipose tissue are known as _____; in obesity, _____ that infiltrate adipose tissue secrete proinflammatory cytokines.

54. Hepatitis _____ virus depends on hepatitis B virus in order to replicate.

55. Jaundice in viral hepatitis occurs during the _____ phase; when jaundice resolves, the _____ phase begins.

56. Cholecystitis occurs when a gallstone lodges in the _____ duct; the most common type of gallstone is made of _____.

57. The primary diagnostic marker for acute pancreatitis is elevated serum _____; chronic pancreatitis is associated with chronic _____ abuse.

58. Fatty liver is associated with chronic use of _____ or with _____ (including in children); although fatty liver is asymptomatic, people who have it may develop steatohepatitis and may progress to _____ or liver cancer.

COMPLETE THE CHART

Compare and contrast Crohn disease and ulcerative colitis by completing this table.

Characteristics	Crohn Disease	Ulcerative Colitis
Family history		
Location of lesions		
Nature of lesions		
Fistulas and abscesses		
Narrowed lumen, possible obstruction		
Recurrent episodes of diarrhea		
Blood in stools		
Clinical course		

MATCH THE RISK FACTORS

Match the cancer on the right with its risk factor(s) on the left.

_____ 59. High-fat diet, inflammatory bowel disease, familial polyposis

_____ 60. Alcohol and tobacco use, reflux

_____ 61. *H. pylori,* high salt intake, nitrates, nitrites

_____ 62. Cirrhosis, chronic hepatitis B or C

A. Esophageal cancer

B. Gastric cancer

C. Primary liver cancer

D. Colon cancer

Write your response to each situation in the space provided.

63. Another nurse asks, "What is the difference between alcoholic hepatitis and alcoholic cirrhosis?"

64. "What is Barrett esophagus?" says Mrs. Cloude. "Is that like heartburn with GERD?"

65. "Why do the enzymes digest the pancreas in pancreatitis?" says Mr. Tran. "I thought the pancreas normally makes those enzymes all the time."

66. "My wife is in ICU, and now she is bleeding from stress ulcers!" says Mr. Wang. "She is unconscious; how can she have stress? I am the one who has stress!"

67. Mr. Higgins had a gastrectomy last year after being diagnosed with gastric cancer. Now he has developed sustained epigastric pain that worsens after eating and is not relieved by antacids. His gastroenterologist diagnosed alkaline reflux gastritis. "My doctor said that I do not have enough stomach left to make a lot of acid," says Mr. Higgins. "What damaged my stomach remnant?"

68. Mr. Jetson has cirrhosis with severe hepatic encephalopathy. His wife says, "I know that my husband's liver is not working well, but how does that cause him to be so drowsy and confused?"

69. A nurse says, "All of our cirrhosis patients have low albumin. How does cirrhosis cause hypoalbuminemia?"

Read the clinical scenario and answer the questions to explore your understanding of ulcerative colitis.

Mary Hawk, age 28, has had episodes of diarrhea and cramping abdominal pain for several months. Recently she developed bloody stools, fatigue, and weight loss.

Family History

Ms. Hawk's mother had ulcerative colitis.

Physical Examination

- Vital signs, cardiac and neurologic examinations normal

- Bowel sounds normal, abdomen flat with mild diffuse tenderness but no rebound tenderness

Laboratory and Diagnostic Tests

- Stool on glove after rectal examination is positive for occult blood

- Complete blood count showed decreased hemoglobin and hematocrit

- Stool sample negative for *C. difficile* toxin, positive for fecal white blood cells

- Colonoscopy reveals inflammation and multiple small bleeding ulcers throughout the rectum and sigmoid colon; biopsy confirmed the lesions to be ulcerative colitis

Ms. Hawk's diagnoses are ulcerative colitis and mild anemia.

70. Inflammatory bowel disease involves genetic predisposition and abnormal (B, T) cell reactions to intestinal (nutrients, microflora).

71. Why did her physician test for rebound tenderness when he examined Ms. Hawk's abdomen?

72. Why is it important to monitor Ms. Hawk's red blood cell count?

73. Why did her physician order a colonoscopy before making the diagnosis?

74. Why was it important to ask Ms. Hawk about her family history of bowel disorders?

75. Why is it important for Ms. Hawk to have periodic colonoscopies to monitor for development of colon cancer?

76. Why should a nurse teach Ms. Hawk to increase her intake of fluid and salt during active episodes of ulcerative colitis?

37 Alterations of Digestive Function in Children

MATCH THE DEFINITIONS

Match each word on the right with its definition on the left.

_____ 1. Chronic scarring of the liver in response to inflammation and tissue damage   A. Atresia

_____ 2. Abnormal narrowing of an opening or lumen   B. Volvulus

_____ 3. Absence of a normal body opening or passageway   C. Stenosis

_____ 4. Twisting of loops of intestine on themselves, which obstructs the lumen   D. Cirrhosis

CIRCLE THE CORRECT WORDS

Circle the correct word from the choices provided to complete these sentences.

5. Neonates who have a congenital anomaly should be examined for the presence of (infection, other anomalies).

6. Children who have (cleft, stenotic) palate tend to have difficulty with (feeding, smiling).

7. In children, chronic hepatitis most often occurs from hepatitis viruses (B and C, A and C); childhood chronic hepatitis usually has (no, numerous) symptoms.

8. In intestinal malrotation, (intussusception, volvulus) can lead to clinical manifestations of bowel obstruction.

9. Stenosis of a segment of bowel causes (collapse, dilation) of the lumen proximal to the obstruction and (collapse, dilation) distal to it.

10. A child who falls below the (third, tenth) percentile on the growth curve is likely to have failure to thrive.

11. A neonate who has meconium ileus should be evaluated for (cystic fibrosis, necrotizing enterocolitis).

12. Rotavirus is a leading cause of (acute diarrhea, necrotizing enterocolitis) in infants and young children.

CATEGORIZE THE CONDITIONS

Write the type of condition beside each name. Choices: congenital, acquired.

_____ 13. Imperforate anus

_____ 14. Esophageal atresia

_____ 15. Hepatitis A

_____ 16. Cleft lip

_____ 17. Tracheoesophageal fistula

_____ 18. Intussusception

_____ 19. Eosinophilic esophagitis

_____ 20. Hirschsprung disease

_____ 21. Cirrhosis

_____ 22. Necrotizing enterocolitis

ORDER THE STEPS

Sequence the events that occur when intussusception occurs.

23. Write the letters here in the correct order of the steps: _____
    A. Constriction of the attached mesentery obstructs venous flow.
    B. Bowel wall becomes ischemic and necrotic.
    C. Proximal intestine telescopes into distal intestine in the direction of peristaltic flow.
    D. Capillaries become engorged, causing edema that compresses arterioles.

EXPLAIN THE PICTURE

Examine the picture and answer the questions about it.

24. This picture shows congenital anomalies. What is the technical name of the anomaly labeled A? _____

25. Why is maternal polyhydramnios associated with this condition?

26. What is the technical name of the anomaly labeled B? _____

27. Given the anatomy of anomaly B, what mechanisms put this infant at high risk for pneumonia?

DESCRIBE THE DIFFERENCES

Describe the difference between each pair of terms.

28. What is the difference between marasmus and kwashiorkor?

29. What is the difference between physiologic jaundice and pathologic jaundice in infants?

MATCH THE RISK FACTORS

Match the condition on the right with its risk factor on the left.

_____ 30. Cleft lip

_____ 31. Distal intestinal obstruction syndrome

_____ 32. Pyloric stenosis

_____ 33. Hepatitis A infection

A. Cystic fibrosis

B. Day-care personnel who do not practice good hand hygiene

C. Maternal smoking or folate deficiency

D. Maternal hypersecretion of gastrin

COMPLETE THE SENTENCES

Write one word in each blank to complete these sentences.

34. Wilson disease is an autosomal _____ defect of _____ metabolism that damages the _____, brain, eyes, and kidneys.

35. In biliary atresia, some of the _____ ducts are absent or obstructed, which leads to development of _____.

36. Gluten-sensitive enteropathy, also called _____ disease, is an autoimmune disease in which autoreactive _____ lymphocytes mediate damage to the intestinal _____.

37. In kwashiorkor, the liver accumulates _____ because of lack of amino acids to make lipoproteins.

38. Children who have marasmus do not have the subcutaneous _____ seen with kwashiorkor, and they have _____ wasting but not edema.

39. Brain damage caused by high bilirubin levels is known as _____.

40. The immature mucosal barrier of a premature infant's gastrointestinal tract is an important factor in the development of _____ _____, which can lead to abdominal distention, _____ perforation, sepsis, and _____.

41. Cystic fibrosis is characterized by deficiency of _____ enzymes, thick respiratory _____, and increased sodium and chloride in _____.

MATCH THE SIGNS AND SYMPTOMS

Match the condition on the right with its typical signs and symptoms on the left.

_____ 42. Chronic constipation, poor weight gain, and progressive abdominal distention; may develop small volume diarrhea

_____ 43. Infant who previously has fed well and gained weight develops repeated forceful vomiting and wants to eat again soon after each vomiting episode

_____ 44. Enlarged spleen, bloody emesis or melena, and ascites

_____ 45. Abdominal pain, bloating, flatulence, and diarrhea after drinking milk

_____ 46. Jaundice, enlarged liver, clay-colored feces, failure to gain weight

A. Portal hypertension

B. Biliary atresia

C. Hirschsprung disease

D. Pyloric stenosis

E. Lactose intolerance

Chapter **37** Alterations of Digestive Function in Children

Write your response to each situation in the space provided.

47. The Endicotts' neonate has meconium ileus and is receiving a therapeutic enema. Mr. Endicott says, "Why does he have meconium rather than a real bowel movement? And why is his meconium so thick?"

48. Travis, age 13 months, had painless rectal bleeding and was diagnosed with Meckel diverticulum. "Why would a little pouch on the intestine bleed?" asks his mother. "And why was that doctor talking about an ulcer?"

49. Diego has been diagnosed with Hirschsprung disease. "I understand that 'megacolon' means big bowel," says his mother. "But what does that other word, 'aganglionic' mean?"

50. Diego's mother has another question about Hirschsprung disease. "But if the bowel contents do not move because the bowel is not contracting, why did Diego have a bit of diarrhea?"

51. Nina has celiac disease. "I understand that we need to avoid gluten in her diet," says her mother, "but I do not understand why Nina did not grow like she should have. A nurse said there was 'flattening of villi' in her intestine, but what does that really mean?"

38 Structure and Function of the Musculoskeletal System

MATCH THE DEFINITIONS

Match each word on the right with its definition on the left.

_____ 1. The narrow tubular portion of a long bone

_____ 2. The broad end of a tubular bone

_____ 3. Substance that gives synovial fluid its viscous quality

_____ 4. Muscle protein that stores oxygen

_____ 5. Connective tissue that attaches muscle to bone

_____ 6. Connective tissue that attaches a bone to another bone

A. Hyaluronate

B. Myoglobin

C. Ligament

D. Tendon

E. Epiphysis

F. Diaphysis

MATCH THE CELL FUNCTIONS

Match each cell on the right with its function on the left.

_____ 7. Secrete hyaluronate into joint fluid

_____ 8. Can differentiate into multiple cell types, including osteoblasts and osteocytes

_____ 9. Help maintain bone by signaling osteoblasts and osteoclasts

_____ 10. Repair or regenerate skeletal muscle

_____ 11. Secrete collagen and other components of cartilage

_____ 12. Lay down new bone

_____ 13. Resorb bone

A. Osteoclasts

B. Chondrocytes

C. Osteoblasts

D. Mesenchymal stem cells

E. Synovial fibroblasts

F. Osteocytes

G. Satellite cells

CIRCLE THE CORRECT WORDS

Circle the correct word from the choices provided to complete these sentences.

14. Spongy bone also is called (compact, cancellous) bone.

15. The small channels that connect the osteocytes in bone are called (lacunae, canaliculi); the spaces in which the osteocytes reside in bone are called (lacunae, canaliculi).

16. In muscle, the greater the innervation ratio of a particular organ, the greater its (speed of contraction, endurance); higher innervation ratios (prevent fatigue, provide precision of movement), and lower innervation ratios (prevent fatigue, provide precision of movement).

17. Ryanodine receptors are located in skeletal muscle (sarcoplasmic reticulum membranes, sarcomere H bands) and are (potassium, calcium) ion channels.

18. With a dynamic (isotonic) contraction, the muscle maintains a constant (length, tension) as it contracts; with a static (isometric) contraction, the muscle maintains a constant (length, tension) as (length, tension) increases.

CATEGORIZE THE SUBSTANCES

For each substance, write its effect on bone resorption beside its name. Choices: inhibits, facilitates.

_____ 19. Osteoprotegerin (OPG)

_____ 20. Prostaglandin E$_2$ (PGE$_2$)

_____ 21. RANKL

_____ 22. Interleukin-6 (IL-6)

_____ 23. Estrogen

_____ 24. Tumor necrosis factor-alpha (TNF-α)

ORDER THE STEPS

Sequence the events that occur in bone remodeling.

25. Write the letters here in the correct order of the steps: _____
    A. Osteoclasts secrete hydrochloric acid and cathepsin K to create resorption cavity.
    B. Osteoblasts lay down layers of bone.
    C. Stimulus activates osteoclasts.
    D. Osteoblasts differentiate into osteocytes.

Sequence the events that occur in bone healing after a fracture.

26. Write the letters here in the correct order of the steps: _____
    A. Osteoblasts form woven bone, known as callus formation.
    B. Fibroblasts, capillary buds, and osteoblasts move into the wound; granulation tissue and cartilage are formed (procallus).
    C. Callus is replaced with stronger bone.
    D. Bone is reshaped through remodeling.
    E. Hematoma forms.

Sequence the events that occur in muscle contraction and then relaxation.

27. Write the letters here in the correct order of the steps: _____
    A. Ryanodine receptors open, and calcium ions flow into the cytoplasm.
    B. Myosin hydrolyzes ATP, and actin–myosin cross-bridges form, causing actin filaments to slide toward myosin filaments, thus shortening the sarcomere.
    C. Muscle fiber action potential spreads along the sarcolemma.
    D. An active transport process moves calcium back into the sarcoplasmic reticulum.
    E. Action potential in motor nerve reaches the neuromuscular junction.
    F. Troponin moves back to its previous position, which closes the actin active sites.
    G. Calcium ions bind to troponin, causing a structural change that opens active sites on actin filaments.
    H. Cross-bridging stops; sarcomeres lengthen.

EXPLAIN THE PICTURES

Examine the pictures and answer the questions about them.

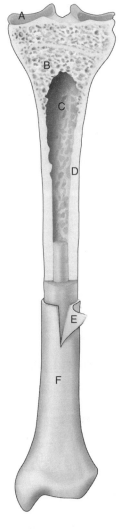

28. The item marked A is _____ cartilage; the major type of collagen it contains is

_____.

29. The item marked B is _____ bone; what substance does its spaces contain?

_____

30. The item marked C is the _____ cavity; what substance does it contain?

_____

31. The item marked D is _____ bone; another name for this type of bone is

_____ bone because it surrounds the other type of bone.

32. The item marked E is the _____; it is made of what type of tissue?

_____

33. The narrow shaft of a long bone, part of which is marked by letter F in the picture, is called

the _____.

34. Which two letters mark locations where osteocytes are found? _____

35. Which letter marks a location where trabeculae are found? _____

36. Which letter marks a location where haversian canals are found? _____

37. Which band in the picture of the striated muscle fiber contains actin? _____

38. Which band contains myosin?

_____

39. Which band will shorten the most when this muscle fiber contracts? _____

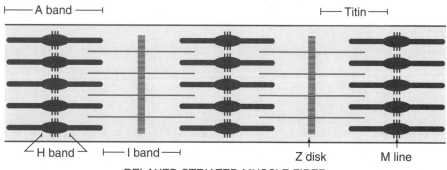

RELAXED STRIATED MUSCLE FIBER

Chapter **38** **Structure and Function of the Musculoskeletal System**

DESCRIBE THE DIFFERENCES

Describe the difference between each pair of terms.

40. What is the difference between compact bone and cancellous bone?

41. What is the difference between a diarthrosis, a synarthrosis, and an amphiarthrosis?

42. What is the difference between osteoid and bone?

43. What is the difference between a synovial joint and a symphysis?

COMPLETE THE SENTENCES

Write one word in each blank to complete these sentences.

44. Members of the transforming growth factor-beta (TGF-β) family are known as _____ _____ proteins because they play important roles in initiation, differentiation, and commitment of precursor cells into _____.

45. Articular cartilage is an organized system of _____ fibers and proteoglycans.

46. The bone directly underneath articular cartilage is called _____ bone; the calcified layer of cartilage that attaches to it is called the _____.

47. The connective tissue framework that surrounds a skeletal muscle is called the _____.

48. An anterior horn neuron, its axon, and the muscle fibers innervated by it are called a _____ _____.

49. Oxygen _____ is the amount of oxygen needed to convert the buildup of _____ acid to glucose and replenish ATP and phosphocreatine stores.

50. Loss of skeletal muscle mass with increasing age is known as _____.

COMPARE AND CONTRAST THE MUSCLE FIBERS

Compare and contrast type I and type II muscle fibers by completing this chart.

Characteristic	Type I Fibers	Type II Fibers
Speed of Contraction		
Intensity of Contraction		
Type of Metabolism		
Number of Mitochondria		
Amount of Myoglobin		
Color		
Capillary Supply		

TEACH PEOPLE ABOUT PHYSIOLOGY

Write your response to each situation in the space provided.

51. A nursing student says, "I know about osteoclasts and osteoblasts, but what are osteocytes?"

52. Jason, a 22-year-old soccer player, says, "If my knee cartilage has no blood supply, how does it get its nourishment?"

53. Ms. Jackson, age 37, says, "What is the difference between striated muscle and skeletal muscle?"

54. A beginning physical therapy student says, "I was so busy memorizing the names of the little tubules that I lost the big picture. Why do muscle fibers need a sarcotubular system?"

55. Mr. Taylor says, "At the gym I hear people talk about building lean body mass. What exactly does that mean?"

56. "A lot of athletes I know are taking creatine supplements for their muscles," says Mr. Young. "What do muscles do with creatine?"

39 Alterations of Musculoskeletal Function

MATCH THE DEFINITIONS

Match each word on the right with its definition on the left.

_____ 1. A break in the continuity of a bone

_____ 2. Failure of broken bone ends to grow together

_____ 3. Inflammation of a tendon where it attaches to a bone

_____ 4. Inflammation in small fluid-filled sacs located between tendons, muscles, and bony prominences

_____ 5. Band of connective tissue that attaches skeletal muscle to bone

_____ 6. Band of connective tissue that connects two bones

A. Bursitis

B. Fracture

C. Tendon

D. Ligament

E. Nonunion

F. Epicondylitis

CIRCLE THE CORRECT WORDS

Circle the correct word from the choices provided to complete these sentences.

7. A (small, substantial) amount of force is needed to dislocate a hip.

8. A tear in a ligament is known as a (strain, sprain); a tear in a tendon is known as a (strain, sprain).

9. A healing tendon or ligament will not be strong enough to withstand a strong pull for 4 to 5 (weeks, months) after injury.

10. Tennis elbow and golfer's elbow are examples of (bursitis, epicondylopathy).

11. Compartment syndromes occur when (venous, arterial) pressure increases, causing eventual ischemia and edema that causes (redness, pain) out of proportion to the injury.

12. Rhabdomyolysis is characterized by (skeletal muscle, chest) pain, weakness, (bloody, dark) urine, and increased serum (creatine kinase, alkaline phosphatase); a main treatment goal is preventing damage to the (liver, kidneys).

13. The most common microorganisms that cause osteomyelitis are (fungi, bacteria); an area of dead bone in osteomyelitis is called (involucrum, sequestrum).

14. In ankylosing spondylitis, an (autoimmune, infectious) process inflames the cartilaginous joints; the primary pathologic problem is uncontrolled bone (destruction, formation), rather than bone (destruction, formation).

15. People who have McArdle disease are unable to (synthesize, break down) glycogen; people who have acid maltase deficiency accumulate glycogen in their (mitochondria, lysosomes).

16. The most common cause of toxic myopathy is (alcohol, autoimmunity).

CATEGORIZE THE CHARACTERISTICS

Write the type of arthropathy beside each characteristic. Choices: osteoarthritis, rheumatoid arthritis.

_____ 17. Subchondral bone sclerosis

_____ 18. Antibodies against citrullinated proteins

_____ 19. Severe joint deformities

_____ 20. Osteophyte formation

_____ 21. Nodule formation in soft tissue

_____ 22. Pannus

_____ 23. Autoimmune disease

_____ 24. Loss of articular cartilage

_____ 25. Joint pain relieved by rest

_____ 26. Joint stiffness for first hour after awakening

ORDER THE STEPS

Sequence the events that occur when a broken bone heals.

27. Write the letters here in the correct order of the steps: _____
    A. Hematoma forms beneath the periosteum around the broken area.
    B. Unnecessary callus is resorbed and trabeculae form.
    C. Osteoblasts in procallus synthesize collagen and matrix, which becomes mineralized into callus.
    D. Necrotic tissue stimulates an inflammatory response.
    E. Vascular tissue invades the fracture area, creating granulation tissue.
    F. Bone-forming cells become activated and produce procallus beneath the periosteum.
    G. Leukocytes release cytokines and other factors that promote healing.

EXPLAIN THE PICTURES

Examine the pictures and answer the questions about them.

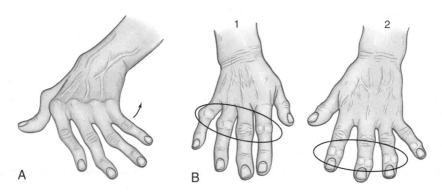

28. What two-word technical term describes the finger deformities in picture A? _____ _____

29. What disease process causes hands to look like picture A? _____

30. In addition to the joint deformities, picture A shows muscle wasting. What caused it?

31. What causes the joint swelling in this condition?

32. Why does this condition have systemic manifestations as well as joint ones?

33. What disease process causes hands to look like picture B? _____

34. The nodes that are circled in hand number 1 are called _____ nodes.

35. The nodes that are circled in hand number 2 are called _____ nodes.

36. What causes these nodes?

37. What is the role of matrix metalloproteinases in this disease process?

MATCH THE FRACTURES

Match each type of fracture on the right with its description on the left.

_____ 38. Fracture with intact skin overlying the bone   A. Linear

_____ 39. Break on only one cortex of bone with splintering of inner bone surface   B. Spiral

_____ 40. Fracture line parallel to long axis of bone   C. Transverse

_____ 41. Fracture with communicating wound between bone and skin   D. Closed

_____ 42. Fracture where bone is weakened by disease   E. Open

_____ 43. Fracture line at an angle (but not perpendicular) to long axis of bone   F. Greenstick

_____ 44. Fragment of bone connected to a ligament or tendon breaks off from the main bone   G. Comminuted

_____ 45. Fracture with one, both, or all fragments out of normal alignment   H. Impacted

_____ 46. Fracture has multiple bone fragments   I. Oblique

_____ 47. Fracture line encircles bone while ascending   J. Displaced

_____ 48. Fracture fragments are pushed into each other   K. Avulsion

_____ 49. Fracture line perpendicular to long axis of bone   L. Pathologic

DESCRIBE THE DIFFERENCES

Describe the difference between each pair of terms.

50. What is the difference between delayed union and malunion?

51. What is the difference between dislocation and subluxation?

MATCH THE PATHOPHYSIOLOGIES

Match each disease on the right with its pathophysiology on the left.

_____ 52. Increased metabolic activity in bone causing abnormal and excessive bone remodeling that enlarges and softens bones

_____ 53. Syndrome involving high levels of uric acid in body fluids, precipitation of urate crystals, and recurrent monoarticular arthritis

_____ 54. Progressive inflammatory changes in shoulder girdle and quadriceps muscles with an autoimmune component

_____ 55. Metabolic disease of adults characterized by inadequate and delayed mineralization of osteoid in mature bone

_____ 5\. Chronic inflammatory joint disease characterized by stiffening and fusion of the spine and sacroiliac joints

_____ 57. Chronic musculoskeletal syndrome characterized by widespread joint and muscle pain, fatigue, and increased sensitivity to touch at tender points

A. Osteomalacia

B. Ankylosing spondylitis

C. Fibromyalgia

D. Paget disease

E. Polymyositis

F. Gout

COMPLETE THE SENTENCES

Write one word in each blank to complete these sentences.

58. Realigning the fragments of a broken bone is called _____; surgical placement of screws, plates, or other devices to immobilize the site is called _____ _____.

59. The term _____ _____ denotes abnormal bone formation in soft tissue that occurs after localized muscle injury.

60. In Paget disease, thickening of the _____ can compress the _____ or cranial nerves.

61. Primary bone cancer is rare, but _____ cancer often affects bone; the most common primary bone cancer in young adults is _____.

62. Classification of bone tumors is based on the cell type and the type of _____ _____ synthesized by the tumor cells.

63. In gout, accumulation of urate crystals in subcutaneous tissue causes formation of white nodules known as _____; precipitation of urate in the kidneys causes renal _____.

64. Failure of a muscle to generate force is called _____; failure of a muscle to sustain force is called _____.

65. Abnormal muscle shortening is called a _____.

66. Tension headaches are due in part to a feedback cycle with the reticular activating system and muscle _____.

67. Chronic fatigue syndrome is characterized by _____ sleep and debilitating fatigue; it is differentiated from fibromyalgia by the absence of _____ points.

68. Prolonged inactivity from bed rest or a cast causes _____ atrophy.

69. Myotonic channelopathies are characterized by delayed muscle _____, whereas an episode of periodic paralysis is characterized by inability to initiate muscle _____.

MATCH THE TUMOR CHARACTERISTICS

Match each tumor type on the right with its characteristic(s) on the left.

_____ 70. Cartilage-forming malignant tumor that does not ossify and grows into surrounding tissue

_____ 71. Benign solitary tumor originating from osteoclasts that is associated with pathologic fractures caused by extensive bone resorption

_____ 72. Malignant bone-forming tumor that typically produces periosteal reaction

_____ 73. Malignant tumor of skeletal muscle that metastasizes rapidly

_____ 74. Collagen-forming solitary malignant tumor that may be a secondary complication of radiation therapy

A. Fibrosarcoma

B. Osteosarcoma

C. Giant cell tumor

D. Chondrosarcoma

E. Rhabdomyosarcoma

TEACH PEOPLE ABOUT PATHOPHYSIOLOGY

Write your response to each situation in the space provided.

75. "The doctor said I have a compound fracture in my leg," says Mr. Reilly. "Does that mean it is infected? I know he is worried about infection."

76. Mr. Tay has osteomyelitis in his lower fibula. He says, "How did my leg bone get infected? The only break in my skin is this oozing diabetes sore on my ankle."

77. Mr. Vargas says, "It has been 3 weeks, and I want this leg cast off now! I have to go back to work! I cannot wait another 3 weeks! My kids are hungry!"

78. "What makes these ugly lumps on my knuckles?" says Mrs. Boult. "The doctor called them Heberden nodes, but he was busy writing prescriptions for my hip arthritis drugs, and I did not ask him."

79. Mr. Crabbe is undergoing treatment for osteosarcoma. He says, "I understand why they do scans to look at my bones, but why do they take blood to monitor bone cancer? Why not just look at the bones?"

CLINICAL SCENARIO

Read the clinical scenario and answer the questions to explore your understanding of osteoporosis.

Mrs. Lottner, age 61, visited a nurse practitioner because she was developing "bent-over posture, just like my mother." History revealed physical inactivity.

Physical Examination

- Vital signs normal except blood pressure 150/88

- Heart and lung sounds normal

- Kyphotic posture

The nurse practitioner ordered a bone mineral density test and repeat blood pressure at a different time. Repeat blood pressure measurements confirmed the diagnosis of hypertension. DXA scan confirmed the diagnosis of postmenopausal osteoporosis.

80. What is the difference between osteopenia and osteoporosis?

81. What relationship between bone formation and bone resorption is responsible for osteoporosis?

82. Why does Mrs. Lottner have a kyphotic posture?

83. At what age did Mrs. Lottner most likely have her peak bone mass? _____

84. What happens to bone mineral density between peak mass and menopause? _____

85. Describe the pattern of change in bone mineral density after menopause.

86. How does lack of estrogen after menopause contribute to osteoporosis?

87. Why did the nurse practitioner encourage Mrs. Lottner to walk every day?

40 Alterations of Musculoskeletal Function in Children

MATCH THE DEFINITIONS

Match each word on the right with its definition on the left.

_____ 1. Bending of the foot downward and forward   A. Equinovarus

_____ 2. Bending of the foot upward and backward   B. Scoliosis

_____ 3. Rotational curvature of the spinal column   C. Dorsiflexion

_____ 4. Clubfoot   D. Plantar flexion

CIRCLE THE CORRECT WORDS

Circle the correct word from the choices provided to complete these sentences.

5. Osteosarcoma commonly is located at the (midshaft, ends) of bones, whereas Ewing sarcoma commonly is located at the (midshaft, ends) of bones.

6. "Corner" metaphyseal fractures are (rarely, almost always) associated with abuse.

7. (Osteomyelitis, Septic arthritis) in children can cause permanent (bone, joint) injury because articular cartilage of (bones, joints) is unable to repair itself after injury from infection.

8. Idiopathic scoliosis is more likely to be severe in (boys, girls).

9. The pathophysiology of Legg-Calvé-Perthes disease occurs at the (tibial tubercle, head of the femur).

10. The pathophysiology of Osgood-Schlatter disease occurs at the (tibial tubercle, head of the femur).

DESCRIBE THE DIFFERENCES

Describe the difference between each pair of terms.

11. What is the difference between osteosarcoma and osteochondroma?

12. What is the difference between osteomyelitis and septic arthritis?

13. What is the difference between septic arthritis and juvenile idiopathic arthritis?

COMPLETE THE SENTENCES

Write one word in each blank to complete these sentences.

14. Infants who have _____ skin folds at the groin should be evaluated for developmental dysplasia of the hip.

15. Idiopathic scoliosis is _____ scoliosis with no known cause.

16. Diseases caused by an insufficient blood supply to growing bones are called _____.

17. The two most common malignant bone tumors of childhood are osteosarcoma and _____ sarcoma; the most common presenting symptom of both cancers is _____.

18. Juvenile idiopathic arthritis that has a severe systemic onset is called _____ disease.

TEACH PEOPLE ABOUT PATHOPHYSIOLOGY

Write your response to each situation in the space provided.

19. A nurse manager of a hospital pediatric unit learns that an 18-month-old boy with osteogenesis imperfecta is being admitted to her unit. What basic facts about osteogenesis imperfecta should the nurse manager teach her staff so that they will give safe care?

20. Alex, age 13, has just been diagnosed with Osgood-Schlatter disease. He says, "Why did part of my tibia die? Will it grow back?"

21. A physician assistant asks, "The father said his 6-month-old baby fell off the sofa. Why did you report suspected child abuse when that baby had a fractured tibia and some bruises? And why did the physician order full body radiographs?"

22. Kiley Norman, age 7 months, had impetigo and developed osteomyelitis. Now she has septic arthritis. Her nurse asks, "Why do infants get septic arthritis with osteomyelitis more commonly than older children do?"

Read the clinical scenario and answer the questions to explore your understanding of muscular dystrophy.

Tommy Lewis, age 3, was brought to a pediatrician's office by his mother, who said, "Tommy is clumsy, falls frequently, and has difficulty climbing stairs."

Physical Examination

- Vital signs normal

- Waddling gait, appears to walk on his toes

- Positive Gower sign

- Calf muscles proportionately larger than other lower extremity muscles

Laboratory Results

- Serum creatine phosphokinase (CPK) level is 14 times normal

- Serum LDH, AST (SGOT), and aldolase all above normal

- Genetic testing confirmed the diagnosis

Tommy's diagnosis is Duchenne muscular dystrophy.

23. Why does classic Duchenne muscular dystrophy occur only in boys?

24. What is the normal function of dystrophin?

25. What is the Gower sign? Why does Tommy have this sign?

26. Why does Tommy have a waddling gait? Appear to walk on his toes?

27. What makes his serum CPK and other enzymes elevated?

28. What caused Tommy's calf muscles to enlarge? Are they strong like hypertrophied muscles?

29. Given his diagnosis, what is the expected clinical course?

41 Structure, Function, and Disorders of the Integument

MATCH THE DEFINITIONS

Match each word on the right with its definition on the left.

_____ 1. Hives
    A. Alopecia

_____ 2. The nail bed
    B. Pruritus

_____ 3. Wart
    C. Urticaria

_____ 4. Infection of a hair follicle; a boil
    D. Hirsutism

_____ 5. The subcutaneous layer of skin
    E. Erysipelas

_____ 6. Hair loss
    F. Furuncle

_____ 7. Itching
    G. Hyponychium

_____ 8. Diffuse bacterial infection of dermis and subcutaneous tissue
    H. Hypodermis

_____ 9. Acute bacterial infection of the upper dermis
    I. Verruca

_____ 10. Excessive hair growth, especially male pattern of hair growth in women
    J. Cellulitis

CIRCLE THE CORRECT WORDS

Circle the correct word from the choices provided to complete these sentences.

11. Sweat glands, sebaceous glands, and hair follicles are located in the (epidermis, dermis).

12. Blood vessels, lymphatic vessels, and nerves are located in the (epidermis, dermis).

13. Blood supply to the skin is regulated by (sympathetic, parasympathetic) nerves to (epidermal, dermal) arterioles.

14. As a person ages, the skin becomes (thinner, thicker), drier, (less, more) elastic, and wrinkled, with (fewer, more) sweat glands.

15. Irritant contact dermatitis (is, is not) mediated by T lymphocytes.

16. Pityriasis rosea may be associated with a (virus, fungus) and begins as a single lesion known as a (rete peg, herald patch).

17. Discoid lupus erythematosus manifests with (skin, systemic) signs and symptoms in genetically susceptible adults, particularly in (men, women) in their late 30s or early 40s.

18. Erythema multiforme produces lesions that look like a target with alternating rings of (edema, necrosis) and (vesicles, inflammation).

19. Lyme disease is caused by a (virus, bacterium) transmitted by (flea, tick) bites.

20. Male-pattern and female-pattern alopecia are similar in that they both involve hair loss in the (frontotemporal, central) area of the scalp, but male-pattern alopecia also includes the (frontotemporal, central) area.

CATEGORIZE THE DISORDERS

Write the type of disorder beside each name. Choices: autoimmune, bacterial infection, viral infection, fungal infection.

_____ 21. Erysipelas

_____ 22. Tinea pedis

_____ 23. Lichen planus

_____ 24. Impetigo

_____ 25. Candidiasis

_____ 26. Alopecia areata

_____ 27. Onychomycosis

_____ 28. Pemphigus

_____ 29. Lupus erythematosus

_____ 30. Psoriasis

ORDER THE LAYERS AND NOTE THEIR FUNCTIONS

Put the layers of the epidermis in order within the table and indicate the function of each layer.

Latin Name of Epidermal Layer	Function of Epidermal Layer
Put the top layer here	

EXPLAIN THE PICTURES

Examine the pictures and answer the questions about them.

Answer the two questions underneath each picture and then identify the lesions.

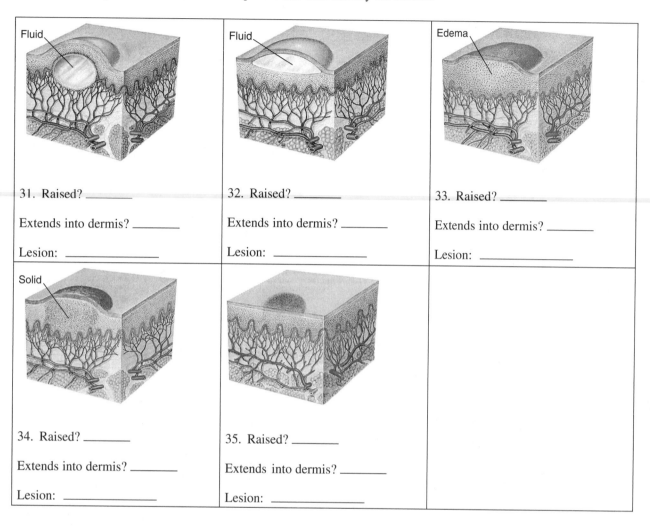

31. Raised? _____

    Extends into dermis? _____

    Lesion: _____

32. Raised? _____

    Extends into dermis? _____

    Lesion: _____

33. Raised? _____

    Extends into dermis? _____

    Lesion: _____

34. Raised? _____

    Extends into dermis? _____

    Lesion: _____

35. Raised? _____

    Extends into dermis? _____

    Lesion: _____

36. How would the picture of the vesicle need to change to make it depict a bulla?

37. How would the picture of the macule need to change to make it depict a patch?

38. The picture from which question number shows a lesion associated with allergic reactions? _____

39. The picture from which question number shows a lesion associated with shingles? _____

DESCRIBE THE DIFFERENCES

Describe the difference between each pair of terms.

40. What is the difference between a furuncle and a carbuncle?

41. What is the difference between apocrine sweat glands and eccrine sweat glands?

42. What is the difference between a hypertrophic scar and a keloid?

43. What is the difference between acne vulgaris and acne rosacea?

MATCH THE FUNCTIONS

Match the cell type on the right with its function(s) on the left.

_____ 44. Provide the barrier function of skin

_____ 45. Process and present antigens to lymphocytes

_____ 46. Secrete pigment that gives color to skin and protects it against ultraviolet radiation

_____ 47. Release histamine; play roles in inflammation and in hypersensitivity reactions in the skin

_____ 48. Secrete the connective tissue matrix and collagen

A. Melanocytes

B. Fibroblasts

C. Keratinocytes

D. Langerhans cells

E. Mast cells

COMPLETE THE SENTENCES

Write one word in each blank to complete these sentences.

49. Many types of skin cancers are associated with damage from _____ exposure, but _____ _____ is associated with herpesvirus type 8.

50. The term _____ can be used interchangeably with the term eczema to describe a particular type of inflammatory response in the skin.

51. Allergic _____ dermatitis from poison ivy is caused by a type _____ hypersensitivity reaction, also called _____ hypersensitivity.

52. Dermatitis that occurs on the legs as a result of chronic venous stasis is called _____ dermatitis; derma-titis that involves scaly, yellowish, inflammatory plaques is called _____ dermatitis.

53. In psoriasis, excessive proliferation of _____ causes abnormal thickened scaly patches of the skin; remissions and _____ are characteristic of psoriasis.

54. In addition to concern about the appearance of their skin, people who have lichen planus are distressed by severe _____.

55. The irreversible bulbous appearance of the nose that occurs in acne rosacea is known as _____.

56. An autoimmune blistering disease known as _____ has several forms, all of which involve _____ against proteins involved in adhesion of the epidermis to the dermis.

57. Candidiasis can occur on the skin, on mucous membranes, and in the _____ _____.

58. Cold sores and genital herpes are caused by the herpes _____ virus, which has two types; although _____ usually causes the cold sores and _____ usually causes genital herpes, either type can cause lesions in either site.

59. The _____ _____ virus causes warts; some strains of this virus predispose to cervical _____.

MATCH THE TUMORS

Match each tumor name on the right with its description on the left.

_____ 60. Benign tumor arising from cutaneous basal cells

_____ 61. Malignant tumor arising from cutaneous basal cells

_____ 62. Benign lesion formed from melanocytes

_____ 63. Malignant tumor arising from melanocytes

_____ 64. Premalignant lesion with aberrant proliferation of epidermal keratinocytes

_____ 65. Malignant tumor arising from the epidermis

_____ 66. Benign tumor arising from hair follicle

_____ 67. Malignant tumor arising from T cells or B cells

A. Nevus

B. Squamous cell carcinoma

C. Cutaneous lymphoma

D. Keratoacanthoma

E. Basal cell carcinoma

F. Malignant melanoma

G. Actinic keratosis

H. Seborrheic keratosis

TEACH PEOPLE ABOUT PATHOPHYSIOLOGY

Write your response to each situation in the space provided.

68. Mrs. Burkhardt says, "Now that I have a lot of gray hair, I would like to know some details of why hair gets gray as we age. Please explain."

Chapter **41** **Structure, Function, and Disorders of the Integument**

69. "My doctor said I have psoriasis. Is that a fungus infection?" says Mrs. Marks. "I am afraid to hug my son because I might give it to him. Is it contagious?"

70. "We are going to take care of my mother at our house when she is released from the hospital," says Mr. Turner. "A nurse told me to make sure she does not lie in one position all day to prevent pressure ulcers. How can lying in a bed cause pressure ulcers?"

71. "I heard that nurse tell the doctor I have wheals on my chest and arms, probably from the penicillin," says Mr. Tier. "They look like hives to me. What is the difference?" Respond directly to him.

72. "My aunt has scleroderma and she doesn't even smile at me anymore," says Agnes Walker, age 11. "Do you think she is mad at me or just sad about having a disease?"

CLINICAL SCENARIO

Read the clinical scenario and answer the questions to explore your understanding of shingles.

Mrs. Maxwell was having financial difficulties during difficult divorce proceedings and was not sleeping well. She was trying to find a second job to support her children and was behind on her rent payments. She developed painful blisters on one side of her chest and went to a nurse practitioner.

Physical Examination

- Vital signs normal

- Reddish wheals on left chest in dermatome distribution (see photo)

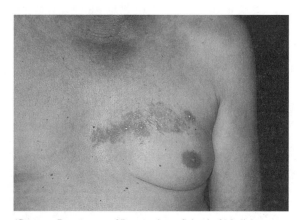

(Courtesy Department of Dermatology, School of Medicine, University of Utah.)

Mrs. Maxwell's diagnosis is shingles.

73. What is the technical term for shingles? _____

74. What virus causes shingles? _____

75. Was this Mrs. Maxwell's first exposure to the virus? Explain your answer.

76. Why do the lesions have this distribution? Why do they not cross the midline?

77. Why might Mrs. Maxwell have developed the shingles now?

78. What condition might persist after the shingles lesions disappear? _____

Chapter **41** **Structure, Function, and Disorders of the Integument**

42 Alterations of the Integument in Children

MATCH THE DEFINITIONS

Match each word on the right with its definition on the left.

_____ 1. A congenital malformation of the dermal capillaries

_____ 2. Fungi that thrive on keratin

_____ 3. Benign tumor formed from rapid growth of vascular endothelial cells that causes formation of extra blood vessels

_____ 4. *Candida* infection in oral mucous membranes

A. Dermatophytes

B. Thrush

C. Port-wine stain

D. Hemangioma

CIRCLE THE CORRECT WORDS

Circle the correct word from the choices provided to complete these sentences.

5. The pathophysiology of atopic dermatitis involves interplay between genetic predisposition, an abnormal (skin, lymphatic) barrier, and dysregulated response of the (endocrine, immune) system.

6. Impetigo is a (mildly, highly) contagious infection of the skin with streptococci or (gonococci, staphylococci); the lesions begin as (macules, vesicles) that rupture to form a honey-colored (crust, ulcer).

7. In staphylococcal scalded-skin syndrome, the toxin (circulates to, is produced in) the skin.

8. Roseola, also known as (herpes zoster, exanthema subitum), causes a (pruritic, nonpruritic) rash that appears (before, after) a high fever, primarily in (infants, adolescents).

9. Hemangiomas tend to (shrink, grow) during the first few years of life and then (shrink, grow).

10. Vascular malformations grow proportionately with the child and (then, do not) regress.

CATEGORIZE THE INFECTIONS

Write the type of infection beside each name. Choices: bacterial, viral, fungal.

_____ 11. Tinea capitis

_____ 12. Impetigo

_____ 13. Thrush

_____ 14. Molluscum contagiosum

_____ 15. Herpes zoster

_____ 16. Tinea corporis

_____ 17. Chickenpox

_____ 18. Measles

Examine the picture and answer the questions about it.

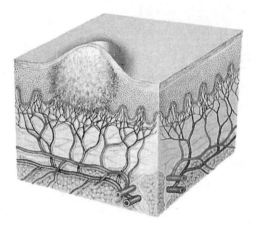

19. This picture shows an acne vulgaris lesion in cross section. What substance fills the lesion?

_____

20. What age group most commonly has this type of lesion?

_____

21. A single acne lesion is a comedo. What is the plural of this term?

_____

22. This lesion is closed at the surface of the skin. Is it a blackhead or a whitehead?

_____

23. Name a type of hormone and a bacterium that contribute to the development of acne.

_____

DESCRIBE THE DIFFERENCES

Describe the difference between each pair of terms.

24. What is the difference between atopic dermatitis and diaper dermatitis?

25. What is the difference between rubeola and rubella?

26. What is the difference between variola and varicella?

27. What is the difference between a strawberry hemangioma and a cavernous hemangioma?

COMPLETE THE SENTENCES

Write one word in each blank to complete these sentences.

28. Children who have atopic dermatitis often have elevated levels of the antibody _____ and a family history of _____ and hay fever, both of which involve this antibody.

29. The technical name for ringworm is _____ _____; this condition is spread by direct or indirect contact with infected people, kittens, or _____.

30. Candida albicans penetrates the epidermal barrier more easily than other microorganisms because it secretes keratolytic _____ and other enzymes.

31. Children who have chickenpox have a risk for developing _____ _____, also known as _____, later in life.

32. Low-flow vascular malformations involve capillaries, _____, and lymphatics; high-flow malformations involve _____.

33. Two blood-sucking parasites are _____, which are nocturnal, and _____, which attach their eggs (also known as _____) to hair shafts.

34. Miliaria rubra, also known as _____ _____, is characterized by erythematous papules associated with excessive _____ in infants.

35. Erythema toxicum _____ is a benign, erythematous accumulation of macules, papules, and pustules that appear at birth or 3 to 4 days after birth and then spontaneously resolve within a few _____.

Chapter **42** **Alterations of the Integument in Children**

MATCH THE CLINICAL MANIFESTATIONS

Match the disorder on the right with its classic signs and symptoms on the left.

_____ 36. Erythematous, round or oval scaling patches that spread
peripherally with clearing in the center, primarily on
nonhairy parts of the face, trunk, and limbs in asymmetric
distribution

A. Impetigo

_____ 37. Acute pruritic vesicles that rupture with a honey-colored
serum and form yellow to white-brown crusts or pustular
lesions

B. Staphylococcal scalded-skin syndrome

_____ 38. Recurrent pruritic red, scaly, crusted lesions on cheeks,
knees, ankles, elbows, or may be more widespread

C. Thrush

_____ 39. Pruritic linear lesions that itch more at night; may also
have vesicles and papules

D. Tinea corporis

_____ 40. Redness and tenderness of skin that becomes widespread,
followed by painful blisters, bullae, and sloughing of skin

E. Scabies

_____ 41. White plaques or spots in the mouth that lead to shallow
ulcers that may bleed when the plaques are removed; may
spread to groin or other areas

F. Atopic dermatitis

TEACH PEOPLE ABOUT PATHOPHYSIOLOGY

Write your response to each situation in the space provided.

42. "My grandson has impetigo," says Mrs. Grey. "What is that? Is it like chickenpox?"

43. "I am not used to working with children," says Nurse Singh. "I need a quick reminder of the characteristics of the rash in chickenpox and in measles."

44. Mrs. Chin says, "If rubella is such a mild illness, why do we vaccinate against it?"

45. Mrs. Dreyer's son Donny, age 6, had a high fever, enlarged cervical lymph nodes, runny nose, and a "barking" cough. She took him to a pediatric nurse practitioner, who told her that Donny probably had measles and would break out in a rash in a day or two. The rash came the very next day. "Donny has measles, just as the nurse practitioner said. All she did was take Donny's temperature, feel his neck, and look carefully in his mouth," says Mrs. Dreyer. "How did she know he had measles?"

Read the clinical scenario and answer the questions to explore your understanding of scabies.

Angie Sherwood, age 11, kept scratching her hands, her armpits, and her elbow creases until her mother took her to an urgent care facility. When asked, Angie reported that the itching is worse at night.

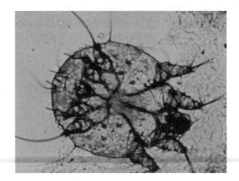

Physical Examination

- Linear erythematous lesions, with a few papules in webs of fingers, elbow creases, and anterior axillary folds
- No other abnormal findings

Laboratory Examination

- Microscopic examination of skin scrapings revealed eggs and an adult mite

Angie's diagnosis is scabies.

46. What causes the linear lesions of scabies?

47. What causes the itching of scabies infestation?

48. What is the major complication of scabies?

49. Why did the physician assistant at the urgent care facility instruct Angie's mother to wash Angie's clothes, bed linen, and towels with hot water and dry them on the hottest cycle, even though they were clean already?

50. Angie's mother says, "Our dog has fleas. Maybe Angie has flea bites instead of scabies. Do the bites look different?" How should the physician assistant respond?

Answer Key

CHAPTER 1

Identify Cellular Structures and Their Functions

1. B; mitochondrion
2. F; ribosome
3. C; Golgi apparatus
4. G; nucleus
5. E; endoplasmic reticulum
6. D; vesicle
7. A; lysosome

Describe the Differences

8. Lysosomes and peroxisomes contain different enzymes. Lysosomes contain digestive enzymes that break down molecules to their component parts, whereas peroxisomes contain oxidative enzymes that are important in producing hydrogen peroxide and other reactive oxygen species.
9. A eukaryote has numerous organelles and a membrane surrounding its nucleus, but a prokaryote does not have organelles, and its genetic material is not organized into a nucleus.
10. A hydrophilic substance attracts water, but a hydrophobic substance repels water.

Match the Definitions

11. D
12. A
13. E
14. B
15. C

Choose the Correct Words

16. G_1
17. differentiation
18. solute
19. oxygen
20. water molecules
21. Paracrine; diffusion
22. the Krebs cycle
23. Active transport
24. proteins

Order the Steps

25. C, A, E, B, D
26. C, B, D, A

Complete the Sentences

27. histones
28. peroxisomes
29. raft
30. fibroblasts
31. hydrostatic
32. isotonic
33. basement
34. Connective
35. muscle

Choose the Direction

36. A
37. B
38. A
39. B
40. A

CHAPTER 2

Match the Definitions

1. I
2. E
3. H
4. F
5. A
6. B
7. D
8. C
9. G

Circle the Correct Words

10. diploid cell
11. single genes
12. males; females
13. DNA
14. amino acids

249

15. triploidy
16. Loss
17. X; females

Describe the Differences

18. Heterozygous means that the two genes at the same locus on both chromosomes are not identical, but homozygous means that the two genes are identical.
19. Monosomy means that one of the chromosomes in somatic cells has only one copy instead of the normal two copies, but trisomy means that one of the chromosomes in somatic cells has three copies.
20. A genotype is an individual's genetic makeup, but a phenotype is the outward appearance of an individual.
21. In mitosis, a diploid cell makes a copy of itself, but in meiosis, a haploid cell is created from a diploid cell.

Order the Steps

22. D, B, E, C, A

Interpret a Pedigree Chart

23. None; the two affected individuals are girls.
24. Mating between two close relatives (consanguineous mating)
25. The symbol for identical twins is:

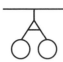

Categorize the Clinical Examples

26. Single-gene disorder
27. Chromosomal disorder
28. Chromosomal disorder
29. Chromosomal disorder
30. Single-gene disorder
31. Chromosomal disorder
32. Single-gene disorder

Complete the Sentences

33. karyotype
34. 23
35. frameshift
36. recessive
37. Alzheimer
38. Klinefelter
39. translocation

Interpret a Punnett Square

40. A

Teach People about Pathophysiology

Compare your answers with these sample answers.

41. We have two copies of most genes. You and Mrs. Medlow each have one PKU gene and one normal gene. PKU is an autosomal recessive disease, which means that a person must have two PKU genes in order to have the disease. You have one PKU gene, so you do not have the disease. Kira has two PKU genes, so she has the disease.
42. *Autosomal* means any chromosome that is not an X or Y chromosome. As you may remember, the X and Y chromosomes are the sex chromosomes. All of the other chromosomes are called autosomal.
43. Yes, cystic fibrosis is autosomal recessive, like PKU. It is caused by a defective gene, and a person must have two copies of the defective gene to have cystic fibrosis.
44. Having two copies of the PKU gene keeps Kira from processing the amino acid phenylalanine, so you manage it by keeping phenylalanine out of her diet. The cystic fibrosis gene makes an abnormal transporter protein in cell membranes, and all of the body's secretions become too thick. That problem cannot be managed with a special diet.

CHAPTER 3

Match the Definitions

1. D
2. A
3. B
4. C

Circle the Correct Words

5. not caused by
6. silencing
7. are
8. imprinting
9. mRNA; miRNA
10. cannot; can
11. twins

Describe the Differences

12. Messenger RNA (mRNA) carries the code for a protein, but noncoding RNA (ncRNA) has regulatory functions.
13. Histones are proteins around which DNA winds, but chromatin is the combination of histones and their associated DNA.
14. Euchromatin is loosely wound so that the genes are accessible for transcription, but heterochromatin is tightly wound so that the genes are transcriptionally inactive.

Complete the Sentences

15. Beckwith-Wiedemann; Russell-Silver
16. promoter
17. oncomirs
18. housekeeping
19. transgenerational inheritance
20. epigenetic

Identify the Enzymes

21. histone acetylases
22. histone deacetylases
23. DNA methyltransferases

Teach People about Pathophysiology

Compare your answers with these sample answers.

24. Hypermethylation silences a gene, so if tumor suppressor genes are silenced, that would encourage development of cancer.
25. You probably learned that messenger RNA carries the genetic code from DNA to the areas of the cell (ribosomes) that make proteins. There are other types of RNAs that do not perform this function. They are called noncoding because they do not carry the genetic code for making proteins. Instead, they participate in other functions, such as regulating which genes become active at any one time.
26. As the cells differentiate, epigenetic silencing of certain genes occurs. The DNA is the same, but some genes are silenced by mechanisms such as DNA methylation. The genes that remain active are the genes that are needed for that particular cell type.

Clinical Scenario

27. Prader-Willi syndrome is caused by a chromosomal deletion on the chromosome 15 inherited from the father. Normally, that section of the gene is read only on the chromosome that is inherited from the father and not on the chromosome inherited from the mother.
28. The genes on the chromosome inherited from the mother are imprinted (transcriptionally silenced). Because those same genes are deleted from the chromosome inherited from the father, no products are produced from those genes during development, causing Prader-Willi syndrome.
29. Imprinting of these genes on the mother's chromosome is normal. The deletion of those genes from the father's chromosome is abnormal.
30. Some of the genes in the deleted region of chromosome 15 that causes both disorders normally are read only from the chromosome inherited from the father; other genes in that region normally are read only from the chromosome inherited from the mother. If the deletion occurs in the chromosome inherited from the father, the child develops Prader-Willi syndrome. If the deletion occurs in the chromosome inherited from the mother, the child develops Angelman syndrome.

CHAPTER 4

Match the Definitions

1. E
2. D
3. G
4. H
5. F
6. B
7. C
8. A

Categorize the Clinical Examples

9. Hyperplasia
10. Hypertrophy
11. Atrophy
12. Metaplasia
13. Hypertrophy
14. Atrophy
15. Hyperplasia

Circle the Correct Words

16. necrosis; apoptosis
17. atypical
18. calcium
19. less; more
20. storage
21. superoxide radicals; membranes
22. do not involve
23. hypoxia; bacterial invasion

Order the Steps

24. B, C, A, E, G, H, F, D

Describe the Differences

25. Hypertrophy increases tissue mass by keeping the same number of cells and making each individual cell larger, but hyperplasia increases tissue mass by increasing the number of cells.
26. Suffocation occurs when oxygen fails to reach the blood, but strangulation occurs when neck pressure collapses blood vessels, stopping blood flow to the brain.
27. An abrasion is a scrape in which superficial skin layers have been removed, but a laceration is a jagged or irregular tearing of tissues.
28. Dystrophic calcification occurs in dying and dead tissues, but metastatic calcification occurs in normal tissues when plasma calcium concentration is too high.

29. With a penetrating gunshot wound, the bullet remains in the body, but with a perforating gunshot wound, the bullet has exited the body.

Complete the Sentences

30. oxygen
31. caseous; liquefactive
32. apoptotic bodies; phagocytosis
33. acetaldehyde
34. oxidative stress
35. somatic
36. melanocytes; keratinocytes
37. caspases

Respond to These Clinical Situations

38. When cells undergo necrosis, enzymes normally found inside cells are released and enter the blood. The enzyme creatine kinase normally occurs inside skeletal muscle. Mr. Martin's injuries caused a lot of skeletal muscle necrosis.
39. After death, when blood no longer is circulating, gravity causes blood to settle in the lowest (most dependent) tissues. Pooling of blood caused the purple discoloration of her skin. That purple discoloration is called livor mortis or postmortem lividity.
40. After death the muscles are relaxed at first, and then they get stiff after several hours.

Draw Your Answers

41.

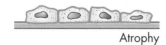

Atrophy

42.

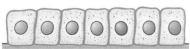

Hyperplasia

Identify the Characteristics

43. B and E

Teach People about Pathophysiology

Compare your answers with these sample answers.

44. Kenesha, when your arm comes out of the cast, it probably will look smaller than your other arm because the cast kept you from using it. When we don't use our muscles, they get smaller and weaker. The good news is that when we do use our muscles, they get bigger and stronger. So if you use your arm again, it can get back to normal size after a few weeks.
45. If you lift weights, your muscles eventually will get bigger and stronger because they are working harder than usual. The same thing happens with the heart muscle if it works harder. Your heart has to work harder than usual to pump against high blood pressure, so your heart muscle got bigger.
46. When the tissue at the ends of your toes died, it was exposed to the air and dried out, making it black and hard. If your Dad's toes were swollen and mushy before they were amputated, they might have been infected. Your blackened toes did not get infected.

CHAPTER 5

Match the Definitions

1. D
2. F
3. A
4. B
5. C
6. E

Circle the Correct Words

7. the same as; freely
8. Albumin
9. osmoreceptors; hypothalamus
10. hypervolemia
11. slow; fast
12. filtration; osmosis
13. carbon dioxide
14. heart

Categorize the Causes of Edema

15. Lymphatic obstruction
16. Increased capillary hydrostatic pressure
17. Increased capillary permeability
18. Increased capillary hydrostatic pressure
19. Decreased plasma oncotic pressure
20. Increased capillary permeability
21. Increased capillary hydrostatic pressure

Select the Greater

22. A lean woman
23. An infant
24. A man
25. A 56-year-old man
26. Intracellular fluid
27. Extracellular fluid
28. The pH of an alkaline solution
29. The respiratory rate during metabolic acidosis

Explain the Pictures

30. hypotonic; hypertonic
31. When the extracellular fluid became hypotonic, the osmolality of the intracellular fluid was greater; osmosis then pulled water into the cell to equalize the osmolalities in the two fluids.
32. Lethargy, confusion, seizures, and coma
33. In both cases, the neurons do not function well. The clinical manifestations are nonspecific indicators of cerebral dysfunction.

Characterize the Hormones

34. E, 2
35. C, 3
36. D, 1
37. A, 5
38. B, 4

Describe the Differences

39. Interstitial fluid is a component of extracellular fluid. Extracellular fluid consists of the fluid inside the blood vessels (intravascular fluid) and the fluid between the cells (interstitial fluid), as well as minor components such as lymph and various secretions (transcellular fluids).
40. A volatile acid (carbonic acid) is excreted by the lungs, but a nonvolatile acid (metabolic acid) is excreted by the kidneys.
41. Acidemia is the state in which the pH of arterial blood is less than 7.35, but acidosis is the condition of having too much acid or too little base, regardless of pH.
42. Correction of an acid-base imbalance returns the bicarbonate and carbonic acid concentrations to normal, but compensation for an acid-base imbalance returns the bicarbonate-to-carbonic acid ratio to normal (20:1) while the actual bicarbonate and carbonic acid concentrations are abnormal.

Complete the Sentences

43. extracellular; intracellular
44. 42
45. edema
46. isotonic
47. respiratory; metabolic
48. 20:1
49. carbonic acid–bicarbonate; hemoglobin
50. acidosis
51. hyperphosphatemia; decrease

Assess the Patients

52. B, 3
53. E, 1
54. D, 2
55. A, 5
56. C, 4

Choose the Direction

57. A
58. A
59. A
60. B

Teach People about Pathophysiology

Compare your answers with these sample answers.

61. Inflammation does cause swelling, but that is not the reason your ankles are swollen. They are not inflamed. They are swollen because your body is overloaded with fluid, and that makes extra outward pressure in your smallest blood vessels. Adding the effects of gravity to that outward pressure makes the swelling appear in your ankles.
62. The location varies with body position. Dependent edema means swelling in the lowermost portion of the body. If your husband has been walking or sitting in a chair with his feet hanging down, then look at his ankles for swelling. If he has been lying on his back in bed all day, then look at the area in the back just above his buttocks.
63. Your body makes metabolic acids from the foods that you eat. That is a normal part of what we call cellular metabolism, the processes by which our cells break down nutrients and use them for energy. You got metabolic acidosis because your body keeps making those metabolic acids, even though your kidneys no longer are able to excrete them. That is why you receive dialysis now.
64. Her fast and deep breathing is her body protecting her from the effects of the ketoacids. When her kidneys could not get rid of the ketoacids fast enough, her breathing sped up to remove another kind of acid called carbonic acid. The important thing to remember is that her fast breathing means that her body is responding normally to protect her, and it is not a lung problem.
65. You can figure out the fluid and electrolyte imbalances in oliguric end-stage renal disease patients if you remember that the kidneys normally excrete water and sodium, potassium, magnesium, phosphate, and metabolic acids. With oliguria, these will not be excreted and will accumulate in the body. Therefore you can expect isotonic fluid excess, hyperkalemia, metabolic acidosis, possibly hypermagnesemia, and hyperphosphatemia.

Clinical Scenario

66. Isotonic fluid deficit. Supporting data: history of diarrhea for 3 weeks, possible orthostatic hypotension (fell when stood up, although muscle weakness might have contributed), tachycardia, weak pulse, low blood pressure when supine, flat neck veins when supine, normal serum sodium.

67. Hypokalemia. Although there are other causes for these manifestations, she has muscle weakness and constipation, which are characteristic of hypokalemia. Hypokalemia also causes orthostatic hypotension.
68. Hypocalcemia and/or hypomagnesemia. Both of these imbalances are caused by decreased intestinal absorption, which could have occurred with her chronic diarrhea; both of them cause muscle cramping, which she has.
69. Metabolic acidosis. Supporting data: history of diarrhea for 3 weeks (loss of bicarbonate in diarrhea), her slowness in responding to questions, and her deep rapid respirations (might be compensation for metabolic acidosis).
70. Isotonic sodium-containing fluid will expand her extracellular fluid volume, which will correct her isotonic fluid deficit. The fluid will replace her deficient electrolytes as well.

CHAPTER 6

Match the Definitions
1. D
2. A
3. B
4. C

Match the Functions
5. C
6. E
7. A
8. B
9. D

Circle the Correct Words
10. anatomic barriers
11. collectins
12. microbiome
13. Defensins; kinins
14. pattern recognition receptors
15. complement; cell lysis

Complete the Overview Table
16. B
17. C
18. A

Categorize the Immune Cells
19. Nonphagocytic innate
20. Adaptive
21. Phagocytic innate
22. Phagocytic innate

Order the Steps
23. B, E, C, D, A, F
24. G, C, A, H, D, B, E, F

Describe the Differences
25. A PAMP is a molecular pattern that is associated with pathogenic microorganisms, but a DAMP is a molecular pattern that is associated with injured or stressed host cells.
26. Opsonins are molecules that mark antigens for destruction by innate immune cells, but cytokines are signaling molecules that influence behavior of immune and other types of cells.

Explain the Pictures
27. Diapedesis
28. They move by chemotaxis to the area where the chemotactic cytokines are in the highest concentration.
29. Polymorphonuclear neutrophil
30. B
31. Macrophages
32. Secrete collagen that forms the scar tissue
33. After

Complete the Sentences
34. innate
35. granuloma
36. cascades
37. keloid
38. dehiscence
39. preformed; synthesizing

Characterize the Exudates
40. C
41. E
42. D
43. B
44. A

Apply Knowledge in Clinical Situations
45. D
46. D
47. A
48. C
49. A

Teach People about Pathophysiology
Compare your answers with these sample answers.

50. Innate immunity is a type of immunity that you have even before you are vaccinated. It is not a specific kind of immunity like a vaccination provides, but it is a general type of immunity. You

have skin to keep out invading microorganisms, innate immune cells that defend against many different microorganisms, and some chemical defenses that help protect you.

51. The red color means your body is taking care of you. When you fell and scraped your knee, the top skin was injured, so your body sent more good red blood to your knee to help fix the injury. The blood brings some helpful clean-up cells that will help your knee get better.

52. When you sprain your ankle, the injured tissue puts out chemical messengers that act on nearby blood vessels. They expand and let more blood flow into the injured tissue, and the blood vessels become leaky. Leaky blood vessels allow fluid from the blood to leak into the tissues, which makes them swell.

53. Yes, white blood cells are in the blood, but when a mosquito bite gets infected, the injured area sends out chemical distress signals. Some of the white blood cells leave the blood and follow the chemical signals, which get stronger the closer they get to the mosquito bite. That is how white blood cells know to come and help get rid of the infection.

54. I think you misunderstood what she said. Nurses use the term *secondary intention* to describe how a pressure ulcer heals. Healing by secondary intention means that the ulcer gradually fills up with new tissue until it heals completely. Healing your ulcer is our first priority for your care, and I know it is your top priority also.

55. The term *normal microbiome* means the good bacteria and other microorganisms that normally live on your skin and in areas of your body like the gastrointestinal tract. These normal microbiome microorganisms help keep disease-causing microorganisms, like that fungus, from causing an infection. When the penicillin killed off some of the normal microbiome, the fungus had an opportunity to grow in their place.

CHAPTER 7

Match the Definitions

1. D
2. E
3. A
4. C
5. B

Complete the Overview

6. <u>B</u> lymphocytes (Humoral), <u>T</u> lymphocytes (Cell-Mediated)

Circle the Correct Words

7. HLA
8. endogenous, exogenous
9. Dendritic cells
10. Th2

Categorize the Clinical Examples

11. Passive
12. Active
13. Active
14. Passive

Order the Steps

15. B, D, E, A, C

Describe the Differences

16. In central tolerance, lymphocytes with receptors against self-antigens are eliminated, but in peripheral tolerance, these cells are suppressed by regulatory T cells and other mechanisms.
17. Antibodies defend against bacteria and viruses, but cytotoxic T cells defend against virus-infected cells and host cells that have become abnormal.
18. MHC class I molecules are located on all nucleated cells and platelets, but MHC class II molecules are located only on antigen-presenting cells, B lymphocytes, and some epithelial cells.

Explain the Pictures

19. A
20. The Fab fragment is the portion that binds the antigen.
21. B
22. Phagocytic innate immune cells bind the Fc fragment with their Fc receptors, which enables them to grasp and phagocytize the antigen that is bound on the other end of the immunoglobulin.
23. The words *antibody titer* indicate that adaptive immunity is involved.
24. Curves in section B
25. Memory cells respond quickly to a previously experienced antigen.

Characterize the Immunoglobulins

26. C
27. D
28. A
29. E
30. B

Complete the Sentences

31. epitope
32. lipid

33. II; I
34. anamnestic
35. cellular; humoral; macrophages; inhibit
36. IgM

Teach People about Pathophysiology

Compare your answers with these sample answers.

37. Antibodies in your blood attach to invading organisms like viruses and bacteria that could make you sick. They help your immune cells to kill the invaders and keep you healthy.
38. Yes, antibodies are proteins, but infants have immature gastrointestinal tracts, and they absorb some proteins whole without their being digested.
39. NK cells are natural killer cells. They do not make antibodies. They attack cells that are infected with virus so that the virus cannot reproduce and spread.

CHAPTER 8

Match the Definitions

1. B
2. D
3. A
4. C
5. F
6. E

Categorize the Organisms

7. Fungus
8. Bacterium
9. Fungus
10. Parasite
11. Fungus
12. Bacterium
13. Fungus
14. Bacterium
15. Parasite
16. Bacterium
17. Bacterium

Circle the Correct Words

18. biofilm
19. Exotoxins; endotoxins
20. capsule
21. avoid recognition by the host
22. sensitized
23. antibodies; cells
24. NK cells
25. autoimmunity
26. donors; no A and B antigens
27. immunocompromised
28. H1
29. only specific

Describe the Differences

30. Epidemic refers to diseases that have a much greater infection rate than usual in a particular population, but pandemic refers to diseases that have a much greater infection rate than usual in a very large area such as a continent or the entire world.
31. Pathogenicity is the ability of an organism to cause disease, but immunogenicity is the ability of an organism to induce an immune response.
32. Primary immune deficiency is congenital, caused by a genetic defect, but secondary immune deficiency is acquired, caused by a condition such as cancer, infection, or normal aging.

Order the Steps

33. B, G, A, F, D, E, H, C
34. I, C, A, E, B, G, F, D, H

Complete the Sentences

35. biofilms
36. pyrogenic
37. disseminated
38. ß-lactamase
39. zoonotic
40. negative; endotoxin
41. self-antigens
42. sensitization
43. B
44. T; thymus
45. activate; block
46. deficiency
47. urticaria

Explain the Picture

48. C
49. They are destroyed in the blood, often by phagocytes.
50. The tissue-bound immune complexes activate the complement cascade, and chemotactic complement fragments (C5a) are produced.
51. Neutrophils bind the Fc ends of the immune complexes, attempting to phagocytize them, and damage the tissue in the process with destructive enzymes and reactive oxygen species.

Teach People about Pathophysiology

Compare your answers with these sample answers.

52. Viruses do reproduce inside cells. However, a virus must reach the cell and attach to it before it can go inside and reproduce. If you have antibodies against a flu virus, the antibodies can bind to the virus outside the cells and keep it from attaching and entering cells. That way the virus will not be able to reproduce and will not make you sick.

53. The term your doctor used is *opportunistic infection*, which does sound a lot like opportunity infection. That means an infection with a microorganism that does not cause infection in people whose immune system is functioning fully but can cause infection in people whose immune system is suppressed like yours. The microorganism seizes the opportunity when the immune defenses are low.

54. The white blood cell soldiers that protect you from measles need to be reminded to do their job from time to time. This shot is a reminder shot. The shot you had when you were a baby caused your white blood cell soldiers to be alert for measles and protect you then, but now you are a big boy and they need a reminder.

55. HIV does destroy CD4+ cells, but right now your body is able to produce them as fast as the virus destroys them. That is why your CD4+ cell count is normal.

56. Nurses follow universal precautions that are expected for all body fluids. Bowel movements can transmit other organisms. If there is blood in the bowel movement, it can transmit HIV, hepatitis B and C, and other blood-borne infections as well.

57. What you have is HIV infection, not AIDS. There is a difference between HIV infection and AIDS. Your positive test tells us that you are infected with the virus but you do not have the low CD4+ cell count or infections that characterize AIDS. You do not have AIDS; you have HIV infection. You can fight your HIV infection by taking the antiretroviral pills that the doctor prescribed. Would you like me to explain these pills to you now?

58. You are correct that phagocytic cells normally dispose of immune complexes when they form. However, in situations when immune complexes are of a certain intermediate size, they are not phagocytized as effectively. Those immune complexes are the ones that deposit in various tissues and cause type III, or immune complex–mediated, hypersensitivity reactions.

59. *Combined* refers to two parts of the immune system that do not work in SCID: the antibody part, also called humoral immunity, and the T lymphocyte part, also called cell-mediated immunity. In some other immunodeficiencies, one or the other of the parts does not work, but because both parts are not working in SCID, it is called a combined immunodeficiency.

60. Calling it a secondary immunodeficiency does not mean that it is unimportant. It means that the immunodeficiency was caused by something outside your immune system, rather than being a problem that started with your immune system. As you know, the cancer drugs suppressed your immunity. That is why

we call it secondary immunodeficiency. We think it is very important also and are working to protect you from infection.

61. It takes 1 to 3 days for any reaction to develop, so we would not see any response in an hour. The type of response that causes a positive test is called a delayed hypersensitivity response because it arises so slowly. It is important for you to have a qualified person look at it later this week. Let us talk about how you can arrange that.

Clinical Scenario

62. The malar rash of SLE commonly is called a butterfly rash because it has the shape of a butterfly with extended wings.

63. Photosensitivity is common with SLE. Her rash is most prominent on sun-exposed areas of her skin.

64. Her elevated BUN and creatinine and urine protein indicate renal dysfunction, which is common with SLE.

65. Remissions and exacerbations of symptoms, arthralgia, pleurisy (pleural friction rub), anemia and mild thrombocytopenia, and positive ANA and anti-DNA antibodies all can occur with SLE.

66. Antinuclear antibodies (antibodies against normal nuclear antigens) are important autoantibodies that participate in the pathophysiology of SLE.

67. SLE is an autoimmune disease, with antibodies against self-antigens causing type III hypersensitivity reactions and other autoimmune processes in many different body tissues.

68. Type III hypersensitivity is an immune complex–mediated reaction in which an antigen–antibody complex lodges in tissue, activating complement, and attracting phagocytes that cause tissue damage.

CHAPTER 9

Match the Definitions
1. C
2. D
3. B
4. A

Identify the Effects of Sympathetic Nervous System Activation
5. Increased
6. Increased
7. Increased
8. Decreased
9. Decreased
10. Increased
11. Increased

Circle the Correct Words

12. nonspecific; Hans Selye
13. leads directly to
14. increases
15. anabolic; catabolic
16. increases; increases
17. uncontrollable

Categorize the Clinical Situations

18. Reactive
19. Reactive
20. Anticipatory
21. Reactive
22. Reactive
23. Anticipatory

Explain the Picture

24. A = corticotropin-releasing hormone (CRH); B = adrenocorticotropic hormone (ACTH); C = cortisol
25. Circles 1 through 4 are + (plus; activating); circles 5 and 6 are – (minus; inhibitory).
26. Negative feedback
27. Circle 4

Identify the Effects of Sleep Deprivation

28. Increases
29. Increases
30. Increases
31. Increases
32. Decreases

Complete the Sentences

33. stress
34. psychoneuroimmunology
35. corticotropin; HPA; sympathetic
36. medulla
37. increased; increased
38. oxytocin
39. cortisol
40. lower (or decrease)

Teach People about Pathophysiology

Compare your answers with these sample answers.

41. The response to stimuli like the sight of an oximeter depends on the individual's perception. An individual who perceives it as a threat will have a stress response, but an individual who perceives it as nonthreatening will not have that response.
42. Immune cells have a lot of receptors in their cell membranes that make them responsive to circulating hormones like epinephrine and to other chemical messengers that increase during the stress response.
43. When we are frightened, our brain turns on the signals that make our heart beat faster and more strongly.

That is a normal response to a scary event. What can I do to help make your chemo less scary? Do you want to watch a video?
44. When you are stressed, your immune cells increase their antibody-making activity and decrease some other activities. That shift in function can make your allergies worse.

CHAPTER 10

Name the Neoplasms

1. E
2. A
3. I
4. G
5. H
6. C
7. B
8. F
9. D

Complete the Chart

Characteristic	Benign Tumors	Malignant Tumors
Appearance of the Cells	Well differentiated	Poorly differentiated
Usual Rate of Growth	Slow	Rapid
Mitotic Index	Low	High
Presence of Capsule	Yes	No
Vascularization	Slight	Neovascularization through angiogenesis
Mode of Growth	Expansile	Invasive
Ability to Metastasize	No	Yes

Circle the Correct Words

10. proto-oncogenes; oncogenes
11. regrow
12. multiple
13. proto-oncogene; oncogene
14. liver
15. heterogeneous
16. oxidative phosphorylation; glycolysis
17. genes; over time
18. Chronic

Match the Definitions

19. E
20. D
21. A
22. C
23. B
24. F

Categorize the Changes

25. Procancer effect
26. Procancer effect
27. Anticancer effect
28. Procancer effect
29. Procancer effect
30. Procancer effect
31. Anticancer effect
32. Procancer effect
33. Procancer effect

Order the Steps

34. B, F, C, A, D, E

Explain the Picture

35. T = Tumor (size and extent of tumor); N = Nodes (lymph node involvement); M = Metastases (extent of distant metastases)
36. Stage
37. T3 N2 M1

Describe the Differences

38. A proto-oncogene is a normal gene that codes for proteins that stimulate cell proliferation appropriately, but an oncogene is a proto-oncogene that is mutated in such a way that its proteins are inappropriately active, accelerating cell proliferation.
39. A proto-oncogene codes for proteins that stimulate cell proliferation, but a tumor suppressor gene codes for proteins that suppress cell proliferation.
40. A driver mutation is important for cancer progression, but a passenger mutation is a random mutation that presumably does not contribute to cancer progression.

Complete the Sentences

41. telomerase
42. angiogenic
43. in situ
44. somatic; germline
45. autocrine
46. inhibition; independence
47. macrophages
48. viral

Teach People about Pathophysiology

Compare your answers with these sample answers.

49. Cancer starts in one location, and then cancer cells can break off and travel to a new location, where they form another tumor, in a process called metastasis. The first place where cancer starts is called the primary tumor. So the cancer in your uncle's body started in his liver. The cancer in your mother's body started in another location, and cells from that primary tumor broke off and moved to your mother's liver. That is why her liver cancer is called metastatic.
50. Some cancers release substances into the blood that cause effects elsewhere in the body. Those effects are called paraneoplastic syndromes. Your husband's cancer cells release a substance called antidiuretic hormone (ADH) into the blood that is causing a paraneoplastic syndrome. Normally, the pituitary gland releases ADH, but feedback controls keep it from making too much ADH. The cancer cells do not have feedback controls, so they keep releasing too much ADH.
51. The Warburg effect describes how cancer cells can metabolize large amounts of glucose rapidly by anaerobic glycolysis to derive their energy for rapid cellular growth. That is different from normal cells that derive most of their energy from aerobic metabolism.
52. No, the reverse Warburg effect does not involve cancer cells making glucose. They need energy to fuel their rapid growth. The reverse Warburg effect involves tumor-associated fibroblasts using anaerobic metabolism to make high-energy chemicals that the cancer cells extract to use for fuel.

Clinical Scenarios

53. Bronchogenic carcinoma arises in the lining of the airways and can cause an obstruction as it grows inward into the lumen.
54. Her cancer arose in her lung. The term *bronchogenic* means that the tumor arose in the bronchi.
55. Obstruction to airflow because of the tumor in the airway and compression of lung tissue from an expanding tumor both can contribute to dyspnea in people who have bronchogenic carcinoma.
56. Repeated exposure to cigarette smoke causes squamous metaplasia in the bronchi, which means that the normal pseudostratified columnar epithelial cells are replaced with squamous cells that can survive more easily in the harsh environment. One or more of these squamous cells eventually accumulated enough mutations to become malignant.

57. Bronchogenic carcinoma frequently metastasizes to the liver.
58. Bronchogenic carcinoma usually does not cause symptoms in its early stages; by the time the cancer is discovered, the tumor may be advanced and there has been time for metastasis to occur.
59. They look at the size of the tumor, how many lymph nodes it has involved, and if it has spread to distant locations in the body.
60. Metastasis. That means the cancer cells have traveled in the blood or the lymph and have formed a new tumor distant from the primary one. The liver is a common place for cancer metastasis.
61. No, cancer can arise in the liver, just as it can arise in the colon. Cancer arises when the genetic material in the cells develops mutations that cause the cells to multiply in an uncontrolled fashion and develop the characteristics of cancer cells.
62. Chemotherapy drugs kill cells that are dividing rapidly. That kills cancer cells, but it also kills some normal cells like the cells in the lining of your mouth. So the drugs that helped get rid of the cancer also made those painful sores. Now that you are no longer receiving chemotherapy, your body has repaired the lining of your mouth.
63. No, chemotherapy drugs usually do not kill red blood cells, but they can kill the rapidly dividing cells in your bone marrow that make the red blood cells. Normally, we make new red blood cells all the time to replace the old ones; during your chemo treatment, you were not making enough new red blood cells. Now that you have recovered, your bone marrow is able to make enough red blood cells.
64. Pain usually does not occur until a cancer is advanced. Your cancer was detected early, before the tumor had grown big enough to put pressure on nerves or cause a lot of tissue destruction and inflammation.

CHAPTER 11

Match the Definitions
1. C
2. A
3. B

Circle the Correct Words
4. silence; methylation
5. immune
6. cigarette smoking
7. decrease
8. xenobiotics
9. anti-apoptotic; increase
10. increases

Categorize the Dietary Factors
11. anticancer
12. anticancer
13. procancer
14. anticancer
15. procancer

Complete the Sentences
16. carcinogens
17. nutrigenomics
18. plasticity
19. decreases
20. adipokines
21. Ultraviolet; basal; melanoma
22. Ionizing
23. Asbestos; radon; water
24. melanoma

Match the Microorganisms
25. B
26. D
27. A
28. C

Teach People about Pathophysiology
Compare your answers with these sample answers.

29. Examples of similar foods to avoid are sausages and meats that are smoked or cured, like bacon. After you eat them, nitrites get changed into chemicals that can damage the genetic material inside your cells and encourage the development of cancer.
30. Actually, drinking a lot of beer can increase your cancer risk. Whether you drink beer or vodka does not matter because both contain alcohol (ethanol, to use the technical word); the alcohol itself is what increases the risk for cancer.
31. The term *bystander effects* does not mean that a person was exposed to radiation. What it means is that cells near the irradiated cells also can be affected, even if they do not receive radiation directly.
32. Transgenerational effects of a carcinogen occur in germline cells, which affects future generations of people. Multigenerational effects involve simultaneous direct exposure of multiple generations to the same carcinogen.

CHAPTER 12

Match the Definitions
1. D
2. A
3. C
4. B

Circle the Correct Words

5. different
6. embryonic
7. rapidly
8. decreased
9. blast

Categorize the Cancers

10. Adults
11. Children/adolescents
12. Children/adolescents
13. Adults
14. Children/adolescents
15. Children/adolescents

Match the Risks

16. D
17. A
18. B
19. C

Complete the Sentences

20. leukemia
21. testicular
22. leukemia
23. Kaposi; lymphoma
24. tumor suppressor

Teach People about Pathophysiology

Compare your answers with these sample answers.

25. Mr. Johnson, it takes a long time for cancer to develop after exposure to the chemicals that are linked to adult cancers. We have not seen strong linkages between environmental chemicals and neuroblastoma in children. Cancers that have the term *blast* in their name arise from immature cells that are unable to mature fully. We are not sure why that happens, but it is very unlikely that chemicals in your home caused your daughter's cancer.
26. Before a baby is born, when it first is growing and developing in the uterus, there are different areas that give rise to different parts of the body. Cancers in children often arise from the area called the mesodermal germ layer. The term *germ* does not mean bacteria or other germs. It means the original place from which the body parts develop.
27. Mr. Talison, your son's diagnosis is not a death sentence. More than 80% of the children who are diagnosed with cancer are cured. Let's talk with your cancer care team and look at the treatment options and the supports that are available for your family.

28. A useful way to think about such studies is the concept of multiple causation etiology. This concept carries the idea that cancer develops because environmental factors interact with predisposing characteristics of the individual. So it is not the pesticides alone that cause leukemia, but the interaction of the pesticides and particular characteristics of the children.
29. Most carcinomas are caused by environmental exposure to carcinogens. Children have not lived long enough to be exposed to carcinogens and subsequent malignant transformation of cells, so childhood carcinomas are quite rare.

CHAPTER 13

Match the Definitions

1. D
2. F
3. J
4. H
5. C
6. A
7. I
8. B
9. G
10. E

Explain the Pictures

11. D
12. B
13. C
14. Axon hillock
15.

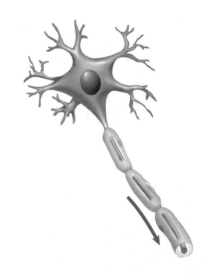

16. Multipolar
17. Node of Ranvier
18. Allows rapid conduction velocity, through saltatory conduction
19. D
20. F
21. Axons
22. Area A is the gray matter, which contains cell bodies of interneurons, and area B is the white matter, which contains tracts of axons, many of which are myelinated.

Circle the Correct Words

23. do not need
24. plasticity
25. divergence
26. potential; real
27. extrapyramidal
28. gray; skeletal
29. sympathetic; parasympathetic
30. sympathetic; postganglionic

Categorize the Physiologic Effects

31. Sympathetic
32. Sympathetic
33. Parasympathetic
34. Sympathetic
35. Parasympathetic
36. Parasympathetic
37. Sympathetic
38. Sympathetic
39. Sympathetic
40. Sympathetic
41. Parasympathetic

Order the Structures

42. A, J, C, G, E, H, F, D, B, I

Match the Functions

43. D
44. F
45. C
46. E
47. A
48. G
49. B

Describe the Differences

50. Efferent nerves carry impulses away from the central nervous system (CNS), but afferent nerves carry impulses toward the CNS.
51. The somatic nervous system consists of sensory pathways and motor pathways that govern voluntary motor control of skeletal muscle, but the autonomic nervous system consists of sensory and motor pathways that regulate primarily involuntary function of body organ systems.
52. A gyrus is a convolution of the cerebral cortex; a sulcus is a shallow groove between adjacent gyri; and a fissure is a deeper groove between adjacent gyri.
53. The cranial nerves arise from the brain and pass through foramina (openings) in the skull, but the spinal nerves arise from the spinal cord and pass through intervertebral foramina of the vertebrae.
54. An excitatory postsynaptic potential (EPSP) is a small depolarization that occurs in a postsynaptic neuron and promotes creation of an action potential, but an inhibitory postsynaptic potential (IPSP) is a small hyperpolarization that occurs in a postsynaptic neuron and inhibits creation of an action potential.

Complete the Sentences

55. 31; cranial
56. neuroglia
57. oligodendroglia; Schwann cells
58. ganglia; nuclei
59. choroid; arachnoid
60. cleft
61. pineal
62. dopamine
63. decussate
64. wallerian; Schwann
65. eyes; tongue; XI

Teach People about Pathophysiology

Compare your answers with these sample answers.

66. Both doctors are correct. The difference is based on how different parts of the brain are connected to the rest of the body. The nerves that come down from the primary motor area of the brain cross over to the opposite side before they communicate to the nerves that tell the muscles what to do. So a stroke that affects the left arm and leg will be in the right side of the brain. On the other hand, the nerves that come from the cerebellum do not cross over but rather stay on the same side. So an injury to the cerebellum that affects coordination on the left side of the body will be in the left side of the cerebellum.
67. Test face for pain, touch, and temperature, using a safety pin and hot and cold objects; test corneal reflex with a wisp of cotton; test motor function of face by asking her to clench her teeth, open her mouth against resistance, and move her jaw from side to side.
68. The names of spinal tracts provide the necessary information. The first part of the name tells where the tract begins. The second part of the name tells where

the tract ends; that is where the axons synapse. So, the rubrospinal tract begins in the red nucleus and goes down the spinal cord; it is a motor tract. The spinothalamic tract begins in the spinal cord and goes to the thalamus in the brain; it is a sensory tract.

69. If his head leans to the side, that could compress a neck vein and increase the pressure in his brain.

CHAPTER 14

Match the Definitions

1. E
2. C
3. F
4. A
5. B
6. D

Circle the Correct Words

7. conduction
8. epinephrine; brown
9. increases
10. higher; lower
11. absence; rapid
12. transduction
13. after

Categorize the Sleep Disorders

14. Dyssomnia; B
15. Parasomnia; C
16. Parasomnia; D
17. Dyssomnia; A

Explain the Picture

18. C
19. Pain sensations from one side of the body go to the contralateral side of the brain. A brain injury in the sensory area on one side of the brain will cause a sensory defect on the opposite side of the body.
20. Paleospinothalamic and neospinothalamic
21. A-delta
22. In the laminae of the substantia gelatinosa in the posterior (dorsal) horn of the gray matter of the spinal cord

Describe the Differences

23. Anosmia is loss of the sense of small, but ageusia is loss of the sense of taste.
24. Conductive hearing loss occurs when sound waves cannot be transmitted through the middle ear, but sensorineural hearing loss occurs when there is defective function of the organ of Corti or its central connections.

25. Strabismus is deviation of one eye from the other when a person is looking at an object, but nystagmus is involuntary rhythmic movement of one or both eyes.
26. Presbycusis is loss of hearing for high-frequency sounds in older adults, but presbyopia is loss of accommodation of the lens of the eye, impairing near vision in older adults.

Complete the Sentences

27. hypothalamus; conservation
28. REM
29. stye; sebaceous
30. REM
31. conjunctivitis
32. optic; increased
33. diplopia; ptosis
34. referred

Teach People about Pathophysiology

Compare your answers with these sample answers.

35. When you exercise, your body generates more heat. Leaving the sweat on your skin while you are exercising is beneficial because it evaporates, removing excessive heat from your body. That is a protection against heat illness. Think of being sweaty during exercise as a sign that you are taking steps to be stronger and healthier.
36. When our immune cells respond to the tissue injury of surgery, they secrete chemicals that we call endogenous pyrogens. These chemicals circulate to the hypothalamus and trigger fever, just like the exogenous pyrogens that you mentioned.
37. Do not worry because he is pale; that is a normal response to a cold body temperature. The body directs blood away from the skin to keep heat from leaving the body. That makes the skin look pale.
38. Glaucoma is too much pressure inside your eye. Although you cannot feel it, that excessive pressure slowly damages your eyes and eventually can cause blindness. You need to use the eyedrops to protect your vision.

Clinical Scenarios

39. Mr. Redd should be positioned flat because he has a decreased circulating blood volume; lying flat will increase perfusion of his brain.
40. He developed heat exhaustion from the interplay of several factors. He was producing heat with physical labor in a hot environment; thermoregulatory mechanisms caused him to sweat profusely, but he was not able to replace the water and salt loss from the sweat, so he became dehydrated.

41. As Mr. Redd's body temperature began to rise, his hypothalamus triggered widespread cutaneous vasodilation. The combination of decreased circulating blood volume and widespread cutaneous vasodilation caused his blood pressure to decrease so that he was not able to perfuse his brain.

42. Tachycardia arose because Mr. Redd's arterial baroreceptors sensed his decreased blood pressure and stimulated his sympathetic cardioaccelerator nerves.

43. Mr. Redd needs to replace his sweat losses with water that has some sodium (salt) in it, such as salty broth or commercial electrolyte replacement fluid. He may tolerate room temperature fluid better than cold fluid at this point.

44. Employee health personnel need to teach Mr. Redd to manage his sweat losses with water and some salt during his workday. They also need to teach Mr. Redd's supervisor the importance of frequent fluid replacement while working in a hot environment and be sure that appropriate fluids are provided in a convenient location.

45. Chronic peripheral neuropathic pain

46. Physiologic adaptation to persistent chronic pain occurs, so the sympathetic nervous system is not highly activated.

47. Neuropathic pain occurs when nerves are damaged. The injured nerves become hyperexcitable and fire in the absence of pain signals from the tissues. On the other hand, nociceptive pain occurs when the free nerve endings of primary pain afferents respond to stimuli from the tissues. In other words, nociceptive pain occurs when the nerves are intact.

CHAPTER 15

Match the Definitions

1. F
2. G
3. A
4. H
5. C
6. D
7. B
8. E

Circle the Correct Words

9. increasing; decreasing; apnea
10. brainstem; nearby
11. greatly
12. vasogenic
13. upper; lower
14. both upper and lower
15. abnormal movement

Categorize the Dysfunctions

16. Hypokinesia
17. Hyperkinesia
18. Hyperkinesia
19. Hypokinesia
20. Hyperkinesia
21. Hyperkinesia
22. Hyperkinesia

Explain the Pictures

23. Flexed; extended
24. Decorticate
25. Cerebral cortex
26. Extended; extended
27. Decerebrate
28. Brainstem (midbrain, upper pons)

Order the Levels of Consciousness

29. D, B, C, F, G, A, E

Describe the Differences

30. Hyperkinesia is excessive movement, but hypertonia is abnormally increased muscle tone.
31. Arousal is a state of being awake, but awareness involves content of thought.
32. Delirium is an acute confusional state caused by dysfunction of neurons and potentially is reversible; dementia is a confusional state caused by death of neurons and is not reversible.
33. Paralysis is loss of voluntary motor function, but paresis is weakness (partial paralysis) of voluntary motor function.
34. Paraplegia is paralysis of both lower extremities, but hemiplegia is paralysis of the upper and lower extremities on one side of the body.

Complete the Sentences

35. status epilepticus
36. focus
37. hydrocephalus
38. stops
39. herniate
40. dominant; involuntary
41. flaccidity; spasticity
42. cerebelli
43. brainstem
44. vegetative

Clinical Scenarios

45. Your husband had a seizure, but that does not mean he has epilepsy. His seizure was caused by low blood sugar. Epilepsy is recurrent seizures for which no underlying cause can be discovered or corrected. He

had one seizure, and we know that his low blood sugar caused it.

46. Generalized seizure. Partial seizures originate in one hemisphere, but generalized seizures involve both hemispheres from their onset.

47. Initial extensor muscle contraction with excessive muscle tone

48. Alternating flexion contraction and relaxation of muscles

49. He was in a postictal state.

50. Extreme muscle contraction during his seizure

51. Neuritic (amyloid) plaques and neurofibrillary tangles. The plaques are collections of fragments of amyloid beta protein that accumulate extracellularly in the brain, disrupt neural transmission, and cause death of neurons. Neurofibrillary tangles are collections of chemically altered tau proteins detached from microtubules that occur intracellularly, disrupt transport processes within the neurons, and also contribute to neuronal death.

52. Many years, even decades

53. Her hippocampus, an area of the brain important for memory and learning

54. Alzheimer disease is progressive, and so far we do not have a way to stop it. The damage is spreading to other parts of her brain, like the part responsible for judgment. We have some resources to help you modify her environment to keep her safe, if you would like them.

55. Forward-flexed (stooped) posture; narrow-based, short-stepped (shuffling) gait that becomes faster as the person walks (festination); loss of postural righting reflexes, muscle rigidity; postural hypotension caused by altered autonomic function and medication side effect; impaired proprioception

56. An extrapyramidal disorder. Motor manifestations are a result of death of dopaminergic neurons that innervate the basal ganglia (the nigrostriatal pathway), causing a deficiency of dopamine and thus altered neurotransmission in pathways that facilitate and inhibit movement.

57. Soft speech is characteristic of Parkinson disease, in part caused by bradykinesia and muscle rigidity that reduce airflow during speech, but also caused by altered sensory perception of the effort expended in vocal production.

58. People who have Parkinson disease, like Mr. Armstrong, have an expressionless face because of muscle rigidity and loss of associated movements caused by their disease. The nonverbal cues that convey emotions are less visible to us. He has a broken hip and says he is in pain; his heart rate, respiratory rate, blood pressure, and blood glucose are elevated, all of which often accompany acute pain. I am sure he needs the pain medication now.

CHAPTER 16

Match the Definitions

1. D
2. C
3. B
4. A

Circle the Correct Words

5. contrecoup; coup
6. venous
7. Infection
8. stretching and tearing
9. mobile
10. unilateral
11. inflammation; impair
12. cervical
13. viruses
14. generalized
15. migraine

Complete the Chart

Function Below the Level of a Complete Spinal Cord Lesion	During the Period of Spinal Shock	After Return of Reflexes
Reflexes	Absent (areflexia)	Present, hyperactive
Motor	Flaccid paralysis	Spastic paralysis
Sensory	Absent	Absent
Bladder	Atonic	Reflex emptying
Bowels	Atonic	Reflex emptying

Draw Your Answers

16.

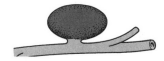

17.

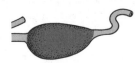

Describe the Differences

18. A brain contusion is a focal bruise that occurs when blood leaks from an injured blood vessel, but a concussion is a diffuse traumatic brain injury.
19. Although both of these conditions can occur after spinal cord injury, mass reflex involves flexor spasms, profuse diaphoresis, piloerection, and automatic bladder emptying, but autonomic dysreflexia involves massive reflex firing of the sympathetic nerves below the level of injury, causing severe hypertension and other sympathetic nervous system manifestations.
20. In myasthenia gravis, a myasthenic crisis is dangerously severe muscle weakness caused by the disease process, but a cholinergic crisis is dangerously severe muscle weakness, diarrhea, intestinal cramping, and other signs of anticholinesterase drug toxicity.

Complete the Sentences

21. epidural (or extradural)
22. consciousness; amnesia
23. excitotoxicity
24. vasogenic; low
25. cerebrovascular
26. pulposus
27. artery
28. tension
29. abscess

Compare the Demyelinating Disorders

Teach People about Pathophysiology
Compare your answers with these sample answers.

30. I know you are worried about Calvin's safety. See how Calvin is responding less and less to you when you try to talk with him? The bleeding above the surface of his brain is squeezing his brain and causing it to function poorly. It can damage his brain unless surgery is done to relieve the pressure.
31. Your brother and your friend have different types of injuries. Your friend has damage to the nerves that go from his spine to his leg muscles. Nerves are like electrical wires that send signals. Your friend's muscles do not get any signals, so they just lie there "flabby-like," as you said, and he cannot move them. Your brother has damage to different nerves: the ones that go down his spine from his brain. That is why he cannot tell his legs to move. However, the nerves that go from his spine to his leg muscles are still working. His legs are spastic because his muscles are getting messages to contract, but those messages are no longer initiated or coordinated by his brain.
32. Multiple sclerosis damages the insulating myelin on nerve cells, and they do not work well. The signs and symptoms of multiple sclerosis are different in different people because the damage can occur many different places in the brain and spinal cord.
33. Severe headache and neck stiffness
34. We have several different kinds of cells in our brains. As you may know, the brain cells that transmit messages are called neurons. The neurons are not making your husband's brain tumor. We have other brain cells called astrocytes because they are somewhat star shaped. The astrocytes are the ones that are reproducing out of control and becoming the tumor. *Oma* means tumor, so his tumor made of astrocytes is called an astrocytoma.

Characteristic	Multiple Sclerosis	Guillain-Barré syndrome
Location of the Demyelinated Axons	Central nervous system	Peripheral nervous system
Pathogenesis of the Demyelination	Genetic predisposition; T cells autoreactive against myelin enter the brain; autoreactive B cells produce autoantibodies; microglial activation and inflammation destroy myelin sheaths, denuding axons	Often triggered by an infection; T cells autoreactive against myelin infiltrate into peripheral nerves; activated macrophages destroy myelin sheaths, denuding axons
Signs and Symptoms	Quite variable, depending on location of lesions; diplopia, paresthesias, motor decrements, urinary and bowel dysfunction	Ascending flaccid paralysis, from feet upward; respiratory muscle weakness may occur; possible sensory changes
Usual Clinical Course	Remissions and exacerbations, with decreasing baseline; or steady declining course	Return of motor function, descending from neck to toes; some people have residual weakness
Cells That Produce Myelin during Remyelination	Oligodendrocytes	Schwann cells

35. Our eyes have muscles attached to them that control how the eyes move. Normally, both eyes are coordinated so that we see only one image because our nerves tell our eye muscles how to work together. The places where the nerves tell the muscles what to do are called neuromuscular junctions. Myasthenia gravis involves abnormal antibodies that change the neuromuscular junctions so that they do not work as well. Therefore your eye muscles become less coordinated and you see double.

Clinical Scenarios

36. Right hemiparesis
37. Left side
38. Ischemic stroke
39. Atrial fibrillation is a risk factor for embolic ischemic stroke because blood clots formed in the left atria can embolize to the brain.
40. Cigarette smoking, obesity, high blood pressure, type 2 diabetes mellitus, and family history of cardiovascular and cerebrovascular disease all are risk factors for thrombotic ischemic stroke because they promote development of atherosclerosis. Rupture of an atherosclerotic plaque in a cerebral artery can trigger formation of a thrombus that occludes the artery.
41. Different areas of the brain control different functions. When a stroke damages part of the brain, that function is impaired. Your husband's stroke damaged the area of his brain that controls voluntary movement of his right arm and leg. His grandfather's stroke damaged another area of his brain: the area that controls speech.
42. Although the signs and symptoms of a TIA do go away, TIAs are a big risk factor for having another stroke. The same changes in your blood vessels that cause TIAs also cause strokes. That is why it is important to protect your blood vessels by taking your blood pressure and other medications, managing your diabetes and your weight, and working to stop smoking. I know these changes are challenging, but they help protect you from another stroke. Your doctor wants to know if you have a TIA so she can help you.
43. Autonomic dysreflexia
44. Greatly elevated blood pressure and bradycardia
45. Uncontrolled reflex activation of sympathetic neurons below the level of injury increases blood pressure by increasing peripheral vascular resistance. Baroreceptor response above the level of injury causes the bradycardia.
46. The extremely high blood pressure could burst an intracerebral artery, causing a hemorrhagic stroke.
47. Sensory stimulation from a distended bladder or rectum, pressure ulcer, wrinkles, or foreign objects under the paralyzed portion of the body
48. Autonomic dysreflexia does not occur with T10 injury because so much of the sympathetic nervous system (SNS) still has supraspinal control with a T10 injury. For autonomic dysreflexia to occur, most of the SNS supraspinal control must be lost.

CHAPTER 17

Match the Definitions

1. C
2. D
3. A
4. B

Circle the Correct Words

5. folate
6. cerebellum; defect of neural tube closure
7. static
8. gait and bladder control; myelomeningocele
9. brain, 1 year
10. motor
11. benign

Characterize the Disorders

12. B, 2
13. C, 1
14. A, 3

Describe the Differences

15. A meningocele is a form of spina bifida in which the meninges protrude but the spinal cord remains in the spinal canal, but myelomeningocele is a form of spina bifida with protrusion of both the spinal cord and meninges through the skin.
16. Pyramidal cerebral palsy is spastic because it involves injury to the pyramidal (corticospinal) pathways, which are upper motor neurons, but extrapyramidal cerebral palsy is nonspastic because it involves damage to basal ganglia or other brain areas that influence involuntary movement and coordination.

Complete the Sentences

17. hemorrhagic
18. hydrocephalus; cerebrospinal
19. bacteria
20. B; birth
21. enzyme; amino; tyrosine
22. absence
23. brain tumor
24. location; growth

Teach People about Pathophysiology

Compare your answers with these sample answers.

25. There are many different types of seizures. The "falling down and twitching all over" type of seizure you described is a generalized seizure and involves the entire surface of the brain. Tim has a different kind called a simple partial seizure. It involves only a

small portion of his brain, so he does not lose consciousness or have that dramatic "twitching all over" type of response. It is, however, a real seizure.

26. Your baby is not paralyzed. He has meningitis, which means that his meninges (the membranes that surround his brain and spinal cord) are inflamed. Have you seen an inflamed finger or ankle? The inflamed part is painful when you try to move it. Baby Hector will not bend his neck because that would stretch his inflamed meninges and would be too painful. Straightening his legs also stretches his meninges so that is why he cried. He will be more willing to move as his meningitis resolves.

27. What you described is normal. Little babies have that cute palmar grasp reflex. As their nervous system matures, the reflex goes away. That normally happens at age 6 months, so your baby is developing normally. See how he responds to your smile now?

28. Hydrocephalus does mean having too much fluid in the brain, a special fluid called cerebrospinal fluid. The pictures you saw of hydrocephalus were little babies who developed hydrocephalus before the bones that form the skull had fused together. When babies are born, the pieces of their skull have not yet fused together, so there is room for their brains to grow. Remember when Jeannie was a baby and she had a fontanel? As she developed, her fontanel went away because her skull bones fused together and became solid. Infants who develop hydrocephalus that is not treated do get great big heads because their skulls can expand from the excess fluid. But when children whose skulls are solid, like Jeannie, develop hydrocephalus, their skulls cannot expand, and the excess fluid inside makes increased pressure that can cause brain damage. That is why the doctors need to work quickly to help Jeannie.

CHAPTER 18

Name the Glands and Their Hormones

1. Gland: pineal; one hormone: melatonin
2. Gland: hypothalamus; six hormones: corticotropin-releasing hormone (CRH), thyrotropin-releasing hormone (TRH), growth hormone–releasing hormone (GHRH), somatostatin, gonadotropin-releasing hormone (GnRH), prolactin-releasing factor (PRF)
3. Gland: pituitary; seven hormones from anterior: adrenocorticotropic hormone (ACTH), melanocyte-stimulating hormone (MSH), thyroid-stimulating hormone (TSH), growth hormone (GH), luteinizing hormone (LH), follicle-stimulating hormone (FSH), prolactin; two hormones from posterior: antidiuretic hormone (ADH), oxytocin
4. Gland: thyroid; three hormones: T_4, T_3, calcitonin
5. Gland: adrenal; three hormones from cortex: aldosterone (mineralocorticoids), cortisol (glucocorticoids),

adrenal androgens; two hormones from medulla: epinephrine, norepinephrine
6. Gland: pancreas (islets); four hormones: insulin, glucagon, amylin, somatostatin
7. Gland: parathyroid; one hormone: parathyroid hormone

Match the Definitions

8. C
9. E
10. D
11. B
12. A

Categorize the Hormones

13. Steroid
14. Peptide
15. Amine
16. Peptide
17. Peptide
18. Steroid
19. Peptide
20. Peptide

Circle the Correct Words

21. a nerve tract; portal blood vessels
22. short; free
23. up-regulate; increases
24. cell membrane
25. proteins
26. GH
27. Lipid; DNA; nucleus
28. ACTH, cortex
29. insulin-like growth factors; somatomedins
30. medulla
31. increases; fight-or-flight response
32. decrease; increase
33. increase; inhibit; numerous
34. negative

Match the Functions

35. C
36. A
37. B
38. E
39. D

Describe the Differences

40. Direct effects of a hormone are changes in cell function that result specifically from stimulation by a particular hormone, but permissive effects are less obvious hormone-induced changes that facilitate the maximal response or functioning of a cell.
41. Autocrine action is a hormone acting on the cell that produced it, but paracrine action is a hormone acting on a nearby cell that it reaches through the interstitial fluid.

42. Negative feedback occurs when the end result of hormone action on target cells suppresses secretion of that hormone, but positive feedback occurs when the end result of hormone action on target cells increases secretion of that hormone.

Complete the Sentences

43. cholesterol
44. vasopressin
45. receptors
46. cAMP
47. hypothalamus
48. thyroid
49. glucagon; amylin
50. thyroid; calcium
51. growth; growth factor
52. posterior; anterior

Teach People about Physiology

Compare your answers with these sample answers.

53. Urine insulin does not give us information about blood insulin levels because most insulin is destroyed in the body by enzymes and not excreted in the urine.
54. A second messenger, like cGMP, is a substance released into a cell when the first messenger reaches the cell and signals it but cannot enter the cell. The second messenger travels inside the cell and triggers cellular chemistry to happen, creating the clinical effects of that first messenger. For example, hormones and other signaling molecules that are small proteins cannot enter cells; they signal the cell from outside, which often causes a second messenger to be released. This is a normal process.
55. Although ADH is released from the posterior pituitary, it is synthesized in areas of the hypothalamus. Apparently his tumor damaged that portion of the hypothalamus, so he cannot make enough ADH.
56. We do make thyroid hormones every day, but then we store large amounts of those hormones in the thyroid glands. So when your new drug stops your thyroid gland from making new thyroid hormones, you still have a lot of stored thyroid hormones that will be released each day. Only after the stored ones are used up will we see the full drug effect.
57. Some hormones, such as ADH and ACTH, are water soluble and do not need carrier proteins in the blood. Thyroid hormones and steroid hormones are not water soluble, so they need carrier proteins.
58. Renin acts on a substance called angiotensinogen that normally circulates in the blood. It converts it to angiotensin I. Then enzymes in the capillaries of the lungs convert angiotensin I to angiotensin II, which stimulates the cortex of the adrenal glands to secrete the hormone aldosterone. Aldosterone circulates to the kidneys and causes them to put more salt and water back into the blood. That kidney action increases the blood volume and can increase the blood flow in the kidney blood vessels.

CHAPTER 19

Match the Definitions

1. B
2. D
3. E
4. A
5. C

Sort the Disorders

6. SIADH; diabetes insipidus
7. Primary hyperthyroidism; primary hypothyroidism
8. Cushing disease; secondary hyperthyroidism; secondary hypothyroidism

Circle the Correct Words

9. high
10. hypersecretion; hyposecretion
11. increased
12. higher
13. 1
14. 1; cytotoxic T lymphocytes
15. amylin; glucagon
16. capillaries; large and medium-sized arteries

Match the Clinical Manifestations

17. F
18. E
19. A
20. H
21. I
22. G
23. J
24. C
25. B
26. D

Describe the Differences

27. A primary endocrine disorder is caused by a problem in the gland that secretes a hormone whose action is directed toward other tissues rather than to another gland, but a secondary endocrine disorder is caused by a problem with a gland that secretes a hormone whose target tissues are another gland that it stimulates or suppresses.
28. Thyrotoxicosis is the effects of having too much thyroid hormone, as seen with hyperthyroidism, but thyrotoxic crisis is the effects of dangerously high levels of thyroid hormone, with high fever, extreme tachycardia, and potential death from heart failure or cardiac dysrhythmias.
29. Neurogenic diabetes insipidus is caused by a problem in the hypothalamus of posterior pituitary that

decreases ADH release, but nephrogenic diabetes insipidus is caused by a problem in the kidney itself that causes insensitivity to ADH.

3 . Acromegaly occurs with hypersecretion of growth hormone in adults, but giantism occurs with hypersecretion of growth hormone in children and adolescents whose epiphyseal plates have not yet closed, so their long bones are able to grow.

Complete the Sentences

31. pheochromocytomas
32. decreased
33. panhypopituitarism
34. anterior; prolactinomas; galactorrhea
35. myxedema; decreased
36. goiter; TSH
37. diabetic ketoacidosis
38. stones
39. disease; syndrome

Explain the Picture

40. Exophthalmos
41. Graves disease (If you answered hyperthyroidism, remember that there are several causes of hyperthyroidism. Exophthalmos is associated specifically with Graves disease.)
42. Exophthalmos occurs when thyroid-stimulating immunoglobulins cause infiltration of fat and other substances that enlarge the contents of the eye socket.

Teach People about Pathophysiology

Compare your answers with these sample answers.

43. People who have type 2 diabetes make a little insulin, which goes to the liver and reduces formation of ketoacids. People who have type 1 diabetes have severe insulin deficiency, and they have excessive fat breakdown and make ketoacids faster than the body can remove them.
44. A child who has too much growth hormone grows tall like a giant, but if an individual already is an adult before developing too much growth hormone, then the effects are different because the long bones have already stopped growing. Adults with growth hormone excess develop enlarged jaw, forehead, and tongue, and large hands and feet, like you noticed with your wife.
45. Your parathyroid glands make parathyroid hormone and send it out into the blood. Parathyroid hormone circulates in the blood to your bones and changes them. The action of parathyroid hormone takes a little calcium out of the bones. Because your body is making too much parathyroid hormone, too much calcium came out of your bones and made them weaker than they should be.
46. That does seem strange, doesn't it? However, there is a very good reason. Your nurses are monitoring for a complication of thyroid surgery that they can detect that way and get treated quickly if it occurs. During thyroid surgery, sometimes the parathyroid glands are injured because they are located right by the thyroid. With parathyroid gland injury, the blood calcium decreases and makes nerves and muscles jumpy and crampy. We can detect low blood calcium in the early stages with the blood pressure cuff as they are doing, so the nurses are taking good care of you.
47. Diabetes insipidus is different from diabetes mellitus, the sugar problem. Diabetes insipidus is a problem with a hormone called antidiuretic hormone, or ADH. ADH tells your kidneys to concentrate your urine. Diabetes insipidus occurs when the kidneys do not receive enough ADH signals. You may have noticed that the nurses are emptying your urine catheter bag very frequently. Your kidneys are making a lot of very dilute urine because ADH is not telling them to concentrate the urine.
48. Fat cells make signaling chemicals and release them into the blood. Some of these signaling chemicals cause your body to be resistant to the action of insulin, the hormone that normally moves sugar into cells. That makes your blood sugar too high. Insulin resistance is part of the problem in type 2 diabetes. If you lose weight, you will have less insulin resistance.
49. Your adrenal gland does not make enough cortisol and aldosterone, two hormones that normally help maintain your circulating blood volume. Without the normal action of these hormones, your blood volume gets too low. When you stand up, gravity pulls your blood downward, and if your blood volume is too low, your brain does not get enough blood to bring it the oxygen it needs. That makes you lightheaded.

Clinical Scenario

50. Insulin resistance and pancreatic beta cell dysfunction
51. All of these factors can contribute to development of gangrene after a minor foot injury: diabetic neuropathy (lack of pain from injury); diabetic retinopathy (more difficult to examine feet); tissue hypoxia from capillary closure in microvascular disease and accelerated atherosclerosis in macrovascular disease; impaired immune function and delayed healing from chronic hyperglycemia; glucose in tissues provides culture medium for pathogens.
52. Retinal cells are highly metabolic and need a good blood supply. Vision loss from diabetic retinopathy is progressive. Initially, microvascular disease from hyperglycemia causes thickening of retinal capillary basement membranes, vein dilation, microaneurysm formation, and hemorrhages. Progression of retinal ischemia causes infarcts with scarring. Eventually, new blood vessels and fibrous tissue form within the retina or optic disc.

53. Microvascular
54. Gastroparesis; autonomic neuropathy; microvascular
55. She is at risk for diabetic nephropathy, which is manifested first by microalbuminuria.
56. Pallor, sweating, tachycardia, palpitations, hunger, anxiety, tremors, fatigue, irritability, decreased ability to concentrate, drowsiness, confusion
57. Polyuria, polydipsia, hypotension, tachycardia, lethargy, confusion, stupor, coma
58. Diabetes speeds up the processes that cause hardening of the arteries, so the heart muscle gets less blood supply. The hardened, narrow arteries to the heart muscle are likely to develop a clot, which cuts off the blood supply and causes a heart attack.
59. In addition to delayed healing if lesions occur, diabetes also causes accelerated atherosclerosis. Atherosclerosis in the femoral arteries creates poor arterial circulation in the lower extremities.

CHAPTER 20

Match the Definitions
1. D
2. F
3. E
4. A
5. B
6. C

Classify the Cells
7. Agranulocyte
8. Agranulocyte
9. Agranulocyte
10. Granulocyte
11. Agranulocyte
12. Granulocyte
13. Granulocyte

Circle the Correct Words
14. do not have; multilobed
15. granulocytes
16. blood cells; bone marrow
17. vascular; osteoblastic
18. four; four; ferrous Fe^{2+}
19. absorption; transferrin; ferritin
20. inhibit; trigger

Match the Functions
21. C
22. F
23. D
24. E
25. G
26. B
27. A

Name the Progenitors
28. Myeloid
29. Lymphoid
30. Myeloid
31. Myeloid
32. Lymphoid
33. Myeloid
34. Myeloid
35. Lymphoid
36. Myeloid

Describe the Differences
37. A leukocyte is a white blood cell of any type, but a lymphocyte is a special type of white blood cell with specific immune functions.
38. Plasma is the liquid portion of blood with its dissolved substances, but serum is plasma minus the clotting factors.
39. A reticulocyte is an immature erythrocyte that has a nucleus, mitochondria, and ribosomes, but an erythrocyte is fully mature and does not have any of these organelles.
40. Ferritin is a protein that binds and stores iron, but apoferritin is ferritin that does not have iron attached.
41. Mitosis is normal cell division that includes DNA replication, anaphase, and cytokinesis, but endomitosis is a type of cell division done by megakaryocyte progenitors in which DNA replication occurs, but anaphase and cytokinesis are blocked, thus producing a cell with a large polyploid nucleus and numerous organelles that fragment into platelets.

Complete the Sentences
42. albumin; neutrophils
43. reversibly; spleen
44. thrombocytes; megakaryocytes; bone marrow
45. erythrocytes; platelets
46. fibrin; plasminogen; liver
47. older

Explain the Picture
48. Erythropoietin
49. kidney; bone marrow
50. Produce more erythrocytes
51. Tissue hypoxia from decreased amount of oxygen in arterial blood
52. When more erythrocytes are present in blood, they carry more oxygen, which relieves tissue hypoxia and thus decreases the release of erythropoietin

Categorize the Substances
53. Antithrombotic
54. Promotes clotting
55. Antithrombotic
56. Antithrombotic

57. Promotes clotting
58. Promotes clotting
59. Antithrombotic
60. Antithrombotic
61. Antithrombotic

Teach People about Pathophysiology

Compare your answers with these sample answers.

62. Those red cells are not in your body any more. Red blood cells live only about 4 months, so the ones that were transfused are gone, and your body has made new red cells.
63. Yes, reticulocytes are immature red blood cells, but they continue to mature in the bloodstream. Your increased reticulocyte count tells us that your bone marrow is making new red cells.
64. Red blood cells need iron to make hemoglobin. They use hemoglobin to carry oxygen from your lungs to the rest of your body. All parts of your body need oxygen to keep functioning. If there is not enough iron in your diet, your red blood cells will not be able to carry enough oxygen.
65. Red blood cells contain a lot of hemoglobin, a substance that enables them to carry oxygen. When red blood cells die, their hemoglobin is taken apart, and a piece of the hemoglobin is changed chemically into bilirubin. Normally, bilirubin travels in the blood to the liver, where it is changed chemically again. So if the man in the mystery story had a lot of red blood cells die suddenly, it makes sense that he would have a lot of bilirubin in his blood.
66. Platelets store these proteins and other substances in granules. That way they can release them very rapidly.
67. Blood clots have a substance called fibrin in them, and our bodies make protective enzymes that chop up the fibrin to dissolve the clot. D-Dimer is a fibrin degradation product, which means that it is a tiny piece of a fibrin clot that a protective enzyme is trying to remove. If D-dimer is elevated in your blood, it can indicate that there is a clot.
68. When a blood vessel is healing, we make special protective chemicals that dissolve the clot slowly and break it up into very tiny pieces. That way there are no large pieces of clot to cause problems.

CHAPTER 21

1. E
2. G
3. A
4. F
5. C
6. B
7. D
8. J
9. N
10. L
11. M
12. I
13. K
14. H

Circle the Correct Words

15. decreases; turbulent
16. macrocytic
17. alcohol
18. highest; decreases
19. relative; absolute
20. parasites; hypersensitivity
21. late; early
22. production; bone marrow; decreases
23. leukocytosis; leukopenia
24. immature
25. clotting

Categorize Anemias by the Appearance of the Erythrocytes

26. Microcytic-hypochromic
27. Normocytic-normochromic
28. Macrocytic-normochromic
29. Normocytic-normochromic
30. Macrocytic-normochromic

Describe the Differences

31. Leukemias are cancers of blood-forming cells, but lymphomas are cancers of lymphatic tissue.
32. A lymphocytic leukemia arises from the lymphoid cell line that normally produces B and T lymphocytes and natural killer cells, but a myelogenous leukemia arises from the myeloid cell line that normally produces granulocytes, monocytes, erythrocytes, and platelets.
33. Splenomegaly is enlargement of the spleen, but hypersplenism is the overactivity of the spleen caused by splenomegaly.
34. Arterial thrombi are composed primarily of platelet aggregates held together by strands of fibrin, but venous thrombi are composed primarily of erythrocytes, greater amounts of fibrin, and fewer platelets.

Match the Abnormalities

35. D
36. C
37. A
38. B

Complete the Sentences

39. -chromic; -cytic
40. recessive; iron
41. heme
42. stem; leukemia
43. iron

44. B; virus; lymphadenopathy
45. Burkitt; B; jaw; virus
46. acute myelogenous leukemia; chronic lymphocytic leukemia
47. infection
48. multiple myeloma
49. Hodgkin lymphoma

Explain the Pictures

50. Glossitis
51. Koilonychia
52. Iron deficiency anemia
53. Pallor but not jaundice. Jaundice occurs with massive hemolysis, not with anemia caused by decreased erythrocyte production.
54. This question can have several correct answers, such as excessive menstrual bleeding, chronic gastrointestinal blood loss, or any other situation in which iron intake is less than iron loss.

Teach People about Pathophysiology

Compare your answers with these sample answers.

55. Ordinarily, red blood cells do not cause clotting, but your body is making so many red blood cells that your blood is too thick, and that makes it more likely to clot.
56. As you know, anemia means that you do not have enough red blood cells. Red blood cells are needed to carry oxygen to our muscles and other areas of the body. With anemia, your body does not have quite enough oxygen and you feel tired.
57. Your body accumulates too much iron, which can damage your liver. Red blood cells have iron in them, so removing some blood on a regular basis removes iron from your body and protects your liver.
58. Bence Jones proteins are pieces of antibodies that are excreted in the urine in multiple myeloma. They are important because they help establish the diagnosis of multiple myeloma and because they can damage the kidneys.
59. Plasma cells are mature B lymphocytes, a type of immune system cell. Their normal function is to secrete antibodies. In plasma cell myeloma, malignant plasma cells secrete entirely too much of one kind of antibody.
60. In acute leukemia, such as the ALL that Knut has, leukemia cells in the bone marrow crowd out the normal cells that make red blood cells, so the bone marrow is not able to make enough red blood cells. As you may know, red blood cells normally carry oxygen to all parts of the body. With too few red blood cells, the muscles and other tissues do not get enough oxygen, which makes Knut tired.
61. You had a different kind of anemia. Menstruating women can develop iron deficiency anemia from losing iron in menstrual blood every month; iron tablets replace the lost iron and cure the anemia. However, your father has anemia from a different cause. His leukemia cells are crowding out the cells that normally make red blood cells in the bone marrow, so he cannot make enough red blood cells. Giving him iron will not help because the cell factories are not working.
62. When you have a sore throat, there is inflammation, and the immune cells that respond to inflammation become activated. They release chemicals that make the lymph nodes where they accumulate get swollen and painful. In Hodgkin lymphoma, the immune cells are gathering in large number in lymph nodes, which makes them swell dramatically, but the immune cells are not activated, and they do not release the inflammatory chemicals that would cause pain.
63. When the body makes white blood cells, they go through several stages. As they mature, we say that they differentiate. A well-differentiated white blood cell is one that is mature. That is a difference between acute and chronic leukemia. In acute leukemia, which you do not have, the white cells are poorly differentiated, which means that they are immature. In chronic leukemia, the kind you have, the white cells are well differentiated, which means that they are mature, although they do not function normally.
64. Normally we have clotting factors that circulate in our blood and make our blood clot when we need to stop bleeding. However, your husband's blood made so many little clots that it used up most of his clotting factors. Now he is bleeding because he does not have enough clotting factors left.
65. ITP stands for some technical words: *immune thrombocytopenic purpura*. I can explain what that means. *Immune* means that your immune system has started destroying your platelets. Sometimes people use the word *idiopathic* instead of *immune* because we do not know exactly why the immune system starts destroying platelets. *Thrombocytopenic* means that your body has too few platelets in the blood. Platelets normally keep people from bleeding inappropriately. Those red dots in your skin are tiny little bleeding spots because you do not have enough platelets. *Purpura* refers to those purple blotches on your skin where a little blood has oozed into your skin. So ITP means that for some unknown reason, your immune system is destroying a lot of your platelets and that you have little spots and discolored areas because of bleeding in your skin. ITP is not contagious because it is an immune system problem, and it is not caused by virus or bacteria.
66. Von Willebrand disease is a coagulation disorder, which means that he will start bleeding if it is out of control. Look for bleeding gums after oral hygiene, oozing or bleeding from injection or catheter sites, bruising after very little pressure, or nosebleeds.

67. Your symptoms are similar because you both have too few platelets in your blood. However, the reasons that you and your son have too few platelets are different. The cancer drugs suppressed your bone marrow, so your bone marrow is not producing enough platelets. Your son's bone marrow is producing enough platelets, but his immune system is attacking them, so they have a shorter survival time.

Clinical Scenario

68. Normally, dietary vitamin B_{12} is released from foods in the stomach and binds to intrinsic factor, a substance secreted by gastric cells. The vitamin B_{12}–intrinsic factor complex is necessary for vitamin B_{12} absorption in the intestines.
69. Mrs. Swenson developed autoantibodies that triggered destruction of parietal cells in her stomach, so the production of intrinsic factor decreased or stopped. Without intrinsic factor, dietary vitamin B_{12} cannot be absorbed. Because vitamin B_{12} is necessary for erythropoiesis, she developed anemia.
70. Macrocytic-normochromic
71. Numbness and tingling are classic manifestations of pernicious anemia because vitamin B_{12} is necessary for normal nerve function. Nerve demyelination and damage from insufficient vitamin B_{12} are progressive and often not reversible.
72. Cobalamin must be continued (at longer intervals) after her vitamin B_{12} blood level is normal because she still cannot absorb dietary vitamin B_{12}.

CHAPTER 22

Match the Definitions

1. B
2. D
3. A
4. C

Circle the Correct Words

5. 2; growth
6. recessive; heterozygous; homozygous
7. 6-12 months of age; is not
8. decreased; hypothermia; hypovolemia
9. painful
10. alpha; beta; thalassemia
11. A

Describe the Differences

12. Hemoglobin A is normal adult hemoglobin with two alpha chains and two beta chains, but hemoglobin S, associated with sickle cell disease, has a valine instead of a glutamic acid at particular point on the beta chains.
13. People who have sickle cell anemia have two copies of the mutated gene (are homozygous) and produce only hemoglobin S, but people who have sickle cell trait have one mutated gene (are heterozygous) and produce a mixture of hemoglobin A and hemoglobin S.

Complete the Sentences

14. sequestration; cardiovascular collapse
15. Cooley; alpha
16. bleeding; joints
17. lymphocytic; lymphoblasts
18. infection; hypermetabolism
19. painless; virus
20. lymphoid

Match the Hemophilias

21. C
22. A
23. B

Teach People about Pathophysiology

Compare your answers with these sample answers.

24. As you know, your son's hemoglobin has an abnormal structure. One of the amino acids in the protein chains is different from normal. When the inside of his red blood cells becomes dehydrated or too acidic or is without oxygen for too long, then the abnormal hemoglobin polymerizes into long strands. These long strands of hemoglobin change the shape of the red blood cell and force it to sickle.
25. When a lot of red blood cells are destroyed in a short time period, as in a hemolytic crisis, the hemoglobin inside them cannot be processed fast enough and a hemoglobin breakdown product called bilirubin accumulates. When bilirubin enters the body tissues that we can see, it makes them look yellow. People who do not have enough red blood cells often look pale, as you expected, but if they have a lot of rapid hemolysis, what we see is the yellow color we call jaundice.

Clinical Scenarios

26. Mrs. Scott developed antibodies against Rh-positive red cells from her first pregnancy. Her antibodies will cross the placenta. If the fetus is Rh-positive, the maternal antibodies will cause hemolysis in the fetus.
27. Mrs. Scott did not have antibodies against Rh-positive red cells when she first became pregnant. Very few fetal erythrocytes cross the placental barrier into the maternal circulation during a normal pregnancy. However, large numbers of fetal erythrocytes do enter maternal circulation when the placenta detaches at childbirth. Mrs. Scott formed the antibodies against Rh-positive red cells after Jacob was born.
28. Baby Ashley's liver and spleen were enlarged because she had hemolysis during her fetal life and erythropoiesis increased at those extramedullary sites.

29. Baby Ashley became jaundiced after she was born because she has Rh-positive red cells and her mother's antibodies against Rh-positive red cells were causing hemolysis. Her immature liver was unable to conjugate the large amounts of bilirubin that result from hemolysis. Buildup of bilirubin in the blood and tissues causes jaundice.
30. During fetal life, unconjugated bilirubin is excreted through the placenta.
31. Kernicterus is accumulation of bilirubin in neural tissues. It causes severe neurologic damage. Baby Ashley is at risk for kernicterus if she does not receive treatment.
32. Jim's platelet count was low because he developed antiplatelet antibodies that bound to his platelets, causing their destruction by phagocytic immune cells. His bone marrow was not able to make new platelets fast enough to replace those that were being destroyed.
33. His erythrocyte count should have been normal because in idiopathic thrombocytopenic purpura, the autoantibodies are specific for platelets.
34. Platelets are necessary for hemostasis. When the platelet count is low, small leaks in capillaries cannot be plugged, and blood seeps into the skin tissues, causing the areas of bruising known as purpura.

CHAPTER 23

Match the Definitions

1. C
2. F
3. A
4. E
5. B
6. D

Match the Functions

7. Right pulmonary artery; B
8. Superior vena cava; D
9. Pulmonary valve; E
10. Tricuspid valve; K
11. Chordae tendinae; G
12. Inferior vena cava; H
13. Interventricular septum; L
14. Mitral valve; J
15. Aortic valve; A
16. Left pulmonary veins; I
17. Left pulmonary artery; F
18. Aorta (aortic arch); C

Circle the Correct Words

19. three; tricuspid; two; mitral
20. more; more
21. vasoconstriction
22. 70%; small

23. calcium
24. more; less
25. thinner; more; veins only
26. media; smooth muscle and elastic fibers
27. stiffening

Select the Faster One

28. SA node
29. AV node
30. Sympathetic nerve firing
31. Blood flow in an arteriole

Categorize the Effects

32. Vasoconstriction
33. Vasoconstriction
34. Decrease
35. Increase
36. Decrease
37. Increase
38. Increase
39. Vasodilation
40. Vasoconstriction

Order the Steps

41. D, B, E, C, A

Explain the Picture

42. Atrial depolarization
43. Contract (atrial systole)
44. From SA node through atrium, AV node, His-Purkinje system, to ventricular myocardium
45. Contracting (ventricular systole)
46. Q wave
47. To prevent backward flow of blood into the atria when the ventricles contract

Describe the Differences

48. The endocardium is the innermost layer of the heart, but the epicardium is the outermost layer of the heart.
49. Systole is contraction of the muscular wall of a cardiac chamber, but diastole is relaxation of it.
50. Angiogenesis is the growth of new capillaries, but arteriogenesis is a new artery branching off from a preexisting artery.
51. Laminar flow has concentric layers of molecules that move parallel to the vessel wall, but turbulent flow has eddy currents that move in whorls, creating more resistance to flow and a less beneficial effect on the endothelium.

Complete the Sentences

52. semilunar; three
53. left; right
54. coronary; right
55. anterior descending; circumflex

56. acetylcholine; cholinergic; norepinephrine; adrenergic
57. calcium
58. intercalated
59. autoregulation
60. thoracic; subclavian
61. vasorum

Calculate the Answers

62. 60 mm Hg
63. 100 mm Hg
64. 3.5 L/min
65. 60%

Sort the Laws

66. Frank-Starling law of the heart
67. Laplace law
68. Poiseuille law

Teach People about Physiology

Compare your answers with these sample answers.

69. The muscle walls are different thicknesses because the two ventricles need to do different amounts of work. Remember that the right ventricle sends blood to the lungs? The lungs are a low-pressure system, and the right ventricle does not have to work very hard to pump blood into the lung blood vessels. Now, think about the work that the left ventricle has to do. It has to pump the blood out to the rest of the body: head, arms, legs, trunk, everywhere except the lungs. The left heart has to work harder because that is a high-pressure system, so it needs to have a thicker muscle.

70. *LAD* means left anterior descending, which is a branch of the left coronary artery. A blockage in the LAD is concerning because that artery supplies blood to much of the interventricular septum and to portions of both ventricles.

71. Troponin is a relaxing protein. You may remember that binding of myosin and actin creates myocardial contraction. When troponin combines with tropomyosin, another relaxing protein, the two of them prevent myosin and actin from binding for a moment, and the myocardium relaxes.

72. Hearts have special cells that actually generate the heartbeat automatically. So even though the nerves are not attached when a heart is transplanted, the heart still continues to beat. If that function continues normally, no pacemaker is needed.

CHAPTER 24

Decipher the Acronyms

1. DVT; Deep venous thrombosis
2. LDL; Low density lipoprotein
3. STEMI; ST elevation myocardial infarction
4. CAD; Coronary artery disease
5. CHD; Coronary heart disease
6. PAD; Peripheral artery disease
7. MVP; Mitral valve prolapse

Match the Definitions

8. G
9. D
10. A
11. B
12. C
13. E
14. F

Circle the Correct Words

15. edema and ulceration
16. pulmonary; systemic
17. compresses; venous distention
18. resistance; increase
19. less
20. no; lifestyle modifications
21. runs between the layers of the wall
22. HDL; LDL
23. an abnormal immune response; streptococci or other organisms
24. a chronic; compress

Explain the Pictures

25. Atherosclerosis
26. Diapedesis into the artery wall
27. Tunica intima
28. Lipid (specifically, oxidized LDL)
29. Foam cell or foamy macrophage
30. Lipids (specifically, oxidized LDL)
31. Migrating into the tunica intima
32. A collagen cap
33. Figure 2 (figure on the right)
34. Fatty streak formation

Categorize the Clinical Manifestations

35. Left heart failure
36. Right heart failure
37. Right heart failure
38. Left heart failure
39. Left heart failure
40. Left heart failure
41. Left heart failure
42. Right heart failure

Describe the Differences

43. A thrombus is a blood clot attached to the endothelium in a blood vessel or cardiac chamber, but an embolus is a blood clot or other bolus of matter circulating in the blood.
44. Primary hypertension has no precisely known cause, but secondary hypertension is caused by another disease process, such as renal disease.

45. In dilated cardiomyopathy, the cardiac chambers are enlarged (have increased diastolic volume), and the myocardium has decreased contractility, but in restrictive cardiomyopathy, the cardiac chambers have decreased diastolic volume because the myocardium is rigid and noncompliant.

46. Valvular stenosis is narrowing of a valve, which impedes the forward flow of blood, but valvular regurgitation is incomplete closure of a valve, which allows blood to leak backward through the valve.

Identify the Risk Factors

47. **H** I S T O R Y
48. P O L **Y** G E N I C
49. **P** O T A S S I U M
50. A G **E**
51. **R** E N I N
52. O B E S I **T** Y
53. M A G N **E** S I U M
54. S **N** S
55. **S** O D I U M
56. C **I** G A R E T T E S
57. A L C **O** H O L
58. **I** N T O L E R A N C E

Complete the Sentences

59. thromboembolus
60. stasis
61. hypertrophy; myocardial infarction
62. malignant; brain
63. orthostatic; 20; 10; falls
64. bacterial; fat
65. atherosclerosis; atherosclerosis
66. ischemia; infarction
67. adiponectin
68. demand; supply
69. scar
70. reperfusion
71. polyarthritis; erythema; pharynx
72. variant; vasospasm
73. unstable

Match the Consequences

74. C
75. D
76. B
77. A

Teach People about Pathophysiology

Compare your answers with these sample answers.

78. What goes on in your head affects your blood vessels and your heart and can raise your blood pressure. In the short term, stress activates your sympathetic nervous system, causing your blood vessels to squeeze tighter and your heart to beat faster. That raises your blood pressure quickly. And, in the long term, your body's responses to stress make your blood vessel lining not work as well, so your blood pressure stays high all the time. The stress in your head can be quite hard on your body. Would you like to hear a little about what stress management involves?

79. An aneurysm is a place in the wall of an artery that is weaker than normal, so that the blood pushes it outward like a balloon. Your husband's aneurysm is in his aorta, a large artery that has a lot of blood flowing through it. They want to operate to fix the aneurysm before it ruptures. If it ruptures, your husband could bleed to death in a short time. Repairing the area of the aneurysm will reduce the risk for its rupturing.

80. The three big causes of clot development are stasis of blood, increased clotting ability, and injury to the inside of a blood vessel. Stasis of blood means that the blood is not moving, such as when it pooled in your legs during your long car ride. Increased clotting ability means that the blood clots more easily than usual, such as when influenced by the estrogen in contraceptives or hormone supplements. And injury to the inside of a blood vessel means that the lining is rough, such as occurs from cigarette smoking.

81. Even though a heart attack affects the heart and a stroke affects the brain, they are related because the underlying problem is a problem called atherosclerosis. Some people call atherosclerosis "hardening of the arteries." As you may know, arteries are blood vessels that carry oxygen and nutrients to the heart, the brain, and other body parts. The lining of arteries is supposed to be smooth, so the blood can travel easily. When a person has atherosclerosis, the linings of the arteries get narrowed and rough. Sometimes a clot develops and stops the blood flow. If that happens in the heart, the person can have a heart attack. If that happens in the brain, the person can have a stroke. Did your doctor talk with you about ways to manage your diet and exercise to reduce your own risk for having a heart attack or stroke?

82. When we exercise, the heart needs to pump more blood than when we are not exercising, to bring oxygen to our muscles. As you know, you have a narrow valve in your heart. That narrow valve limits the amount of blood that your heart can pump out to the rest of your body. When you are not exercising, your heart is able to pump out enough blood to meet your needs. However, when you exercise, that narrow valve prevents your heart from pumping the extra blood to your muscles and the rest of your body. You get so tired because your muscles are not receiving the extra oxygen they need. And you can get faint when your heart is not able to pump enough blood to your brain.

83. As you may know, your heart muscle contracts to pump blood around your body, and then it relaxes to fill with blood that it will pump out in the next contraction. Heart failure with reduced ejection fraction means that your heart has difficulty emptying when it contracts to pump out the blood. Heart failure with preserved ejection fraction means that a heart does not fill properly when it relaxes.

84. Big strong muscles need more oxygen than normal-sized ones. Abnormally big strong heart muscles may not get enough oxygen through the little blood vessels that serve the heart muscle. When a portion of the heart muscle needs more oxygen than the blood vessels are able to provide, the stage is set for a heart attack to occur.

85. It may or may not be a heart attack. The chest pain and other symptoms he had could be caused by a heart attack or by a blood vessel in his heart squeezing shut temporarily. So they call it "acute coronary syndrome" until they can determine the difference. Meanwhile, they do emergency procedures that can help his heart no matter which of the two problems it is.

86. Your grandma is not having an emergency. Let me explain. You probably saw a TV show on which somebody had *ventricular* fibrillation and it was an emergency. That is a different kind of fibrillation. Your grandma has *atrial* fibrillation. Fibrillation means a muscle is quivering or contracting in a disorganized fashion. Some little muscles at the top of your grandma's heart quiver from time to time and get disorganized, but the rest of your grandma's heart can work without them. Would you like me to draw you a picture of atrial fibrillation?

Clinical Scenarios

87. Ask him about the following: family history of heart disease; personal history of hyperlipidemia, hypertension, diabetes, hyperhomocysteinemia, or atherosclerotic disease in other vascular systems (e.g., history of stroke or peripheral vascular disease); history of cigarette smoking, habitual amount of physical activity, usual diet, and any recent stressors.

88. He may have peripheral vascular disease caused by atherosclerosis.

89. An ECG taken now may be completely normal because his pain (and his transient ischemia) has resolved. It may reveal evidence of previous myocardial infarction.

90. Stable angina is the angina pain from myocardial ischemia that occurs predictably with exertion and is relieved with rest or nitroglycerin.

91. Yes, you are remembering well. Some people experience angina pain in the back, jaw, or shoulder or down their left arm. The chest pain that you experienced is the classic type of angina, but people now realize that myocardial ischemia can cause atypical symptoms also.

92. Cutting down on saturated fat is a great idea because it will reduce one of the risk factors for atherosclerosis. Remember that atherosclerosis in your coronary arteries is the underlying reason for your angina. LDL cholesterol from the saturated fat accumulates in the inner layer of blood vessels and is an important part of an atherosclerotic plaque. If you eat less saturated fat, you reduce your risk. Would you like me to arrange a consultation with a dietitian to help you plan specific ways to eat less saturated fat?

93. He had extracellular fluid volume (ECV) excess. Evidence includes the pulmonary edema and his underlying congestive heart failure, which is known to cause ECV excess. Treatment with diuretics and low-salt diet are appropriate for ECV excess.

94. They heard the adventitious sounds caused by fluid in the alveoli.

95. He likely had bilateral ankle edema caused by increased capillary hydrostatic pressure.

96. He most likely had a bounding pulse.

97. He needs to monitor for increasing ECV excess in order to take action before pulmonary edema arises. A sudden weight gain of 2 pounds (1 kg) indicates a gain of 1 liter of fluid.

98. Sodium holds water in the extracellular fluid, thus expanding the ECV. He needs to reduce his ECV rather than expand it.

CHAPTER 25

Decipher the Acronyms

1. ASD; Atrial septal defect
2. PDA; Patent ductus arteriosus
3. VSD; Ventricular septal defect

Circle the Correct Words

4. 8th
5. cyanosis
6. rarely
7. ventricular; will

Characterize the Congenital Heart Defects

8. E, 2
9. H, 3
10. D, 1
11. C, 3
12. B, 2
13. G, 1
14. A, 1
15. F, 3

Complete the Sentences

16. high; low
17. cyanotic
18. atrioventricular; Down
19. hypoplastic

20. right; left; extrauterine
21. truncus arteriosus
22. Kawasaki; coronary
23. renal
24. hypertension

Teach People about Pathophysiology

Compare your answers with these sample answers.

25. The aorta is a big blood vessel that brings blood from the heart to the rest of the body. That scary word *coarctation* simply means that there is a narrow part in the aorta in the location where there was a passageway before your baby was born. The narrow part of the aorta makes the blood pressure high in your baby's arms and low in his legs, so that is why the nurses are measuring blood pressure in his leg. His leg is fine; the nurses are monitoring the effects of his heart problem.

26. When your baby cries or when she tries to nurse, she needs more oxygen because she is using her muscles. The defects in her heart make less oxygen in her blood, so she does not have enough oxygen when she uses her muscles. The blue color tells us that her muscles need more oxygen than her blood is carrying. She does not nurse very long because her muscles need more oxygen and get tired, not because she doesn't like you. See how her fingers start to curl around your finger when you put it in her hand?

27. Before a baby is born, the ductus arteriosus is a normal blood vessel; you are remembering well. The ductus is supposed to close after birth. The word *patent* means that the ductus arteriosus still is open; because of that, some blood moves abnormally through it between two blood vessels.

28. Your baby has only one heart defect. An atrial septal defect is an abnormal opening between the two top parts of the heart. Blood flowing through that opening is turbulent and makes a sound we call a murmur. Would you like to listen to it through my stethoscope?

29. The reason for the difference in the signs and symptoms is the type of blood that goes out the aorta: with a right-to-left shunt, that blood is not fully oxygenated; with a left-to-right shunt, the blood in the aorta is fully oxygenated, but an extra volume of blood passes through the lungs, causing extra work for the heart. Therefore signs and symptoms of a congenital heart defect involving a right-to-left blood shunt are caused by hypoxemia and cyanosis; they include poor feeding, poor weight gain, dyspnea on exertion, fatigue, and exercise intolerance. By contrast, signs and symptoms of a congenital heart defect that causes a left-to-right blood shunt are caused by pulmonary overcirculation or acyanotic heart failure; they include poor feeding, failure to thrive, dyspnea, tachypnea, orthopnea, and frequent respiratory infections.

CHAPTER 26

Match the Definitions
1. I
2. A
3. H
4. E
5. F
6. G
7. B
8. C
9. D

Order the Steps
10. E, C, G, B, D, A, F, I, H

Match the Functions
11. B
12. D
13. A
14. C

Circle the Correct Words
15. two; three
16. lower
17. veins; arteries
18. oxygenated; left
19. $Paco_2$
20. brainstem
21. constrict; dilate
22. external
23. water vapor; $[(760 - 47) \times 0.209]$
24. Bohr

Explain the Picture
25. Pao_2
26. Sao_2
27. Peripheral
28. Left; increased affinity of hemoglobin for oxygen enables erythrocytes to load up with oxygen in the lungs.
29. Right; decreased affinity of hemoglobin for oxygen enables erythrocytes to release oxygen in the tissues.
30. Decreased pH, increased $Paco_2$, and increased heat from cellular metabolism
31. Left

Describe the Differences
32. A terminal bronchiole is a conducting airway, but a respiratory bronchiole is a gas-exchange airway.
33. Type I alveolar cells provide the structure of alveoli, but type II alveolar cells secrete surfactant.
34. The visceral pleura covers the lungs, but the parietal pleura lines the thoracic cavity.
35. Pao_2 is the partial pressure of oxygen in the arterial blood, but Pao_2 is the partial pressure of oxygen in the alveoli.

36. Ventilation is movement of air into and out of the lungs, but respiration is exchange of oxygen and carbon dioxide during cellular metabolism.

Complete the Sentences

37. upper
38. macrophages
39. respiratory; alveolar; alveoli
40. alveolocapillary
41. 500
42. irritant
43. downward; increasing; negative
44. elastic
45. decreased; increases; increasing
46. 0.8; less
47. Pao_2

Match the Zones

48. C
49. B
50. A

Teach People about Physiology

Compare your answers with these sample answers.

51. Cilia are tiny hairlike structures that beat rhythmically and move a layer of mucus upward toward your throat. That mucous layer traps dust and microorganisms that could make you sick and carries them away from your lungs.
52. A small amount of the blood carried by the pulmonary veins is deoxygenated blood from the bronchial circulation, which is part of the systemic circulation. The bronchial circulation nourishes tissue in the conducting airways and does not participate in gas exchange.
53. When a small bronchiole gets blocked, the alveolar partial pressure of oxygen decreases in the alveoli that airway serves. It is not useful to perfuse alveoli that are not ventilated, so the pulmonary arterioles constrict in that area, sending the blood to other alveoli that are well ventilated. That makes the lungs more efficient.
54. Carbon dioxide diffuses across membranes much more easily than oxygen. That makes it possible to excrete enough CO_2 from the lungs even when a lung problem decreases diffusion of oxygen into the blood.

CHAPTER 27

Match the Definitions

1. D
2. E
3. A
4. B
5. C
6. F

Circle the Correct Words

7. $Paco_2$
8. effusion
9. decreased
10. swallowing; pneumonitis
11. dullness; crackles; pink frothy
12. exudative; transudative
13. nonproductive; low-grade
14. restrictive; obstructive
15. expiration
16. chronic
17. cigarette smoking; vague

Categorize the Causes

18. Hyperventilation
19. Hypoventilation
20. Hypoventilation
21. Hyperventilation
22. Hypoventilation
23. Hyperventilation
24. Hypoventilation

Order the Steps

25. D, C, A, F, B, H, E, G

Explain the Picture

26. asthma
27. No, not the first antigen exposure, as demonstrated by the presence of antigen-specific antibodies (IgE)
28. The IgE is produced by plasma cells (mature B lymphocytes that have become committed to a specific antigen).
29. The mast cell degranulates when antigen binds to the IgE located on the mast cell membrane. Mast cell degranulation releases inflammatory mediators that cause inflammation, bronchoconstriction, and increased mucous secretion.

Describe the Differences

30. Dyspnea is a feeling of breathlessness, but orthopnea is a feeling of breathlessness when lying flat.
31. Absorption atelectasis is alveolar collapse caused by gases being absorbed from alveoli that are obstructed, but compression atelectasis is alveolar collapse caused by external pressure on the alveoli.
32. In a communicating pneumothorax, the pressure of the air in the pleural space is the same as barometric pressure because the air drawn into the pleural space during inspiration is forced back out during expiration, but in tension pneumothorax, the pressure of the air in the pleural space exceeds barometric pressure because air enters during inspiration but cannot exit during expiration.

Match the Breathing Patterns

33. C
34. E

35. D
36. B
37. F
38. A

Complete the Sentences

39. paroxysmal nocturnal dyspnea
40. inward; flail
41. air
42. bronchiectasis; sputum
43. connective (or fibrotic); decreased
44. remodeling
45. mucus; constriction
46. status asthmaticus
47. α_1 antitrypsin; proteolytic enzymes
48. chronic bronchitis; mucus; productive
49. barrel; dyspnea
50. right; hypertension
51. hoarseness
52. bronchogenic carcinoma; hormones

Teach People about Pathophysiology

Compare your answers with these sample answers.

53. Your grandpa has a chronic lung disease called emphysema. Some of the lung structure inside his chest has been destroyed, so he has to use his respiratory muscles extra hard to move air in and out of his lungs.
54. *ARDS* means acute respiratory distress syndrome or adult respiratory distress syndrome. Do you know what inflammation is? If you skin your knee, it gets red and swollen because it is injured, and we call that inflammation. Your uncle has a lot of inflammation inside his lungs, which is making them stiff, so that it is difficult to breathe. That is why he is in the hospital where they are taking care of him.
55. Your cousin may not cough up blood. He breathed in the germs that cause tuberculosis, but his protector white blood cells probably are attacking and surrounding them, so they cannot hurt his lungs badly enough to make him cough blood. It is important for him to take his tuberculosis medicine every day to help get rid of the germs so that he will not cough up blood.
56. While he was working in the coal mine every day, your grandpa breathed in a lot of coal dust. The coal dust went into his lungs, and over the years, his body made scar tissue. Have you seen a scar develop after someone gets a cut? That is what happened deep inside your grandpa's lungs. More and more scar tissue formed until his lungs got very stiff and it is hard for him to breathe.
57. Your relatives were exposed to different kinds of materials in their occupations. Silica is inorganic, which means that it did not come from living material. On the other hand, mold is organic, which means that it is living material. Long-term exposure to both of these materials causes buildup of scar tissue in the lungs that we know as pulmonary fibrosis. However, the actual process that causes that fibrosis is different. Exposure to inorganic materials causes the disease process known as pneumoconiosis; exposure to organic materials causes the disease process known as hypersensitivity pneumonitis.
58. Normally, blood that goes through the lungs and picks up oxygen empties into the left side of the heart, which pumps the blood to the rest of the body. If the left side of the heart is not able to pump out the blood effectively, blood will back up into the blood vessels in the lungs. That makes too much pressure in those lung blood vessels, so some water moves out of the blood vessels and into the lung spaces. He had difficulty breathing because some of his lung spaces had water in them instead of air.

Clinical Scenarios

59. Empyema is pus (white blood cells and bacteria) in the pleural space.
60. Empyema fluid usually originates as leakage of lymphatic drainage from sites of bacterial pneumonia.
61. Mrs. Beeson is short of breath because the accumulated empyema fluid is compressing her left lung or at least preventing it from expanding, which interferes with ventilation and gas exchange.
62. Tuberculosis is transmitted through the air, contained in droplet nuclei created when a person who has untreated active tuberculosis coughs.
63. A tubercle is an accumulation of white blood cells, mostly derived from neutrophils, macrophages, and lymphocytes, around a foreign body or microorganisms that phagocytes are unable to remove effectively.
64. Yes, Mrs. Goh should have had a positive tuberculin test when she had latent TB disease. This test indicates that her immune system has encountered the TB bacillus and reacted to it. It does not distinguish between latent infection and active disease.
65. Mrs. Goh likely developed some sort of immunocompromise. Although there are many possibilities, common causes of immunocompromise include immunosuppressive drugs (e.g., prednisone or cancer chemotherapy), AIDS, or conditions such as chronic alcoholism or liver disease.
66. Low-grade fever, shortness of breath, productive cough, unintentional weight loss of 15 pounds in 4 months
67. Bacterial pneumonia because she has exudate in her alveoli, a productive cough, and a substantial fever and chills, which characterize a bacterial pneumonia. Viral pneumonia usually is mild and self-limited and does not produce a substantial alveolar exudate.

68. Cigarette smoking compromises the upper airway defenses. Bacteria reach the lung, causing inflammation. Bacteria, white blood cells, cytokines, and exudate flood the alveoli, causing V/Q mismatching that leads to hypoxemia.

69. Phagocytic cells, such as macrophages, will clear much of the consolidated exudate.

70. Smoking paralyzes the cilia, can cause squamous metaplasia, can trigger chronic inflammation in the bronchi, and increases the production of mucus. These effects of smoking all compromise the upper airway defenses, making her more vulnerable to pneumonia.

71. Ms. Silber developed a pulmonary embolism from a deep venous thrombosis in the lower extremity that had the fracture.

72. Although ventilation (V) occurs with a pulmonary embolism, a pulmonary embolus stops perfusion (Q) in pulmonary blood vessels, creating ventilation-perfusion (V/Q) mismatch.

73. You could not move your broken leg because it is in a cast, so the blood did not flow very fast in it. Slow-moving blood clots rather easily, which allowed a blood clot to form in one of your deep leg veins. When the clot broke loose, it traveled in the blood to your lungs and got stuck in one of the blood vessels in your lungs. As you probably know, the blood needs to travel through the lungs to pick up oxygen. When the clot blocked blood flow in your lung, you needed more oxygen. That is why you became short of breath and were breathing so fast. [Note: If you used technical terms such as *immobility, stasis of blood, thrombus, embolus, perfusion,* or *ventilation* in your answer without explaining them, remember that you need to use language suitable for a layperson and try your answer again.]

CHAPTER 28

Match the Definitions

1. D
2. C
3. A
4. B

Circle the Correct Words

5. barking
6. bacterial; 2 to 7
7. unilateral; tonsillitis
8. viral
9. atypical; not
10. follows; progressive; hypoxemia

Categorize the Respiratory Disorders

11. Upper airway infection
12. Lower airway infection
13. Upper airway infection
14. Lower airway infection
15. Upper airway infection
16. Upper airway infection

Explain the Picture

17. D
18. A
19. Obstruction in area E will alter the nature of the cough.
20. Stridor
21. Stridor is inspiratory in area B and expiratory in area C.
22. Area A

Complete the Sentences

23. respiratory distress syndrome
24. croup; virus; subglottal
25. adenotonsillar
26. surfactant; hyaline
27. bronchopulmonary dysplasia; development
28. respiratory syncytial virus; rhinorrhea; increased
29. pneumonitis
30. hygiene

Teach People about Pathophysiology

Compare your answers with these sample answers.

31. Croup is swelling inside the neck that makes a little child cough, make strange noises when breathing, and have difficulty breathing. It must have been scary to see and hear that with your little brother. Little children are the ones who get croup. You are too grown up to get croup.

32. Snoring is common with a condition called obstructive sleep apnea. That is an important cause of being sleepy during the day like Jason is.

33. I understand that you are concerned about Howie. The good news is that SIDS happens only in children who are younger than 12 months old. Howie will not develop SIDS because he has grown past the vulnerable age. You will feel more rested and enjoy Howie more during the day if you do not wake yourself up every 2 hours all night.

34. We really do need to remove it now. If it stays in your airways, you could get an infection there. Or it could cause more irritation and swelling that could block your breathing. Your wheezing tells us that your airway already is narrowed now, so we need to pay attention.

35. Dog germs do not cause asthma. Your little sister got asthma because she is likely to have an allergy in her breathing tubes. When she plays with dogs, she breathes in little bits from the dog hairs that trigger her asthma. Apparently, you are not likely to have an allergy in your breathing tubes, so those little bits from the dog hairs do not make you cough and have trouble breathing.

Clinical Scenarios

36. The admitting nurse did not make a mistake. When a child has acute epiglottitis, examination of the throat can trigger laryngospasm, which blocks breathing and may be fatal.

37. Darrell was drooling because the swollen epiglottis was preventing him from swallowing.

38. Turbulent airflow through a partially obstructed airway causes stridor. Darrell's airway was partially obstructed by his swollen epiglottis.

39. The epiglottis is a little flap that normally covers the opening to our airway when we swallow. The epiglottis sends the food or liquid to our stomach when we eat or drink and keeps it from going toward our lungs. *Epiglottitis* means that the epiglottis is inflamed and swollen. Darrell's epiglottis was swollen and blocking his breathing. That is why we put the tube down his throat so that he can breathe.

40. Darrell is unable to swallow, so he was given intravenous antibiotics.

41. Acute epiglottitis that is treated appropriately usually resolves after a few days.

42. CF is an autosomal recessive disorder, which means that a person must have two CF genes in order to have CF. Each of your parents has only one CF gene, so they do not have CF. You inherited one CF gene from each of your parents, which gives you two CF genes.

43. *CFTCR* means cystic fibrosis transmembrane conductance regulator, a protein that transports chloride ions across epithelial cell membranes. A defect in this gene causes cystic fibrosis by creating an abnormal CFTCR that works ineffectively.

44. Factors that contribute to the recurrent respiratory infections in CF include the very thick dehydrated mucus from abnormal CFTCR function that impedes normal mucociliary clearance of bacteria; chronic infection with bacteria that form biofilms; and eventual development of bronchiectasis, which makes pouches where mucus collects and bacteria grow.

45. Chronic infiltration of neutrophils in CF contributes to inflammation through secretion of oxidants (which promote inflammation) and neutrophil elastase and other proteases (which damage tissue and contribute to development of bronchiectasis).

46. Biofilms in the airways in CF enable bacteria to evade the immune system and resist antibiotics.

47. Digital clubbing

48. The CFTCR defect in CF also causes digestive secretions, especially those from the pancreas, to be abnormally thick, which impedes absorption of nutrients.

CHAPTER 29

Match the Definitions

1. C
2. D
3. A
4. F
5. B
6. E

Circle the Correct Words

7. cortex
8. external
9. protein; concentrate
10. excretion
11. glomerular filtration rate
12. increase; decreases; increases
13. low; high; reabsorption
14. uromodulin; distal; bacteria
15. increases; concentrate
16. loop of Henle; vasa recta
17. activate; parathyroid hormone
18. glomerular filtration rate; renal blood flow

Locate the Structures

19. Renal cortex
20. Renal medulla
21. Renal cortex
22. Renal cortex
23. Renal medulla
24. Renal medulla
25. Renal medulla
26. Renal cortex
27. Renal cortex
28. Renal cortex

Order the Steps

29. A, E, G, B, F, H, J, D, I, C

Match the Functions

30. C
31. E
32. B
33. A
34. D

Explain the Picture

35. Proximal convoluted tubule
36. Mitochondria provide ATP for the active transport processes that enable the reabsorption function of these cells.
37. Microvilli increase the surface area for reabsorption.
38. The cell of the thick ascending limb of the loop of Henle

Match the Mechanisms

39. B
40. C
41. A

Describe the Differences

42. The urethra carries urine from the bladder to the exterior of the body, but a ureter carries urine from the kidney to the bladder.
43. The principal cells secrete potassium and reabsorb sodium and water, but the intercalated cells reabsorb potassium and secrete hydrogen ions.
44. Tubular secretion moves substances from the peritubular capillaries into the renal tubular lumen, but tubular reabsorption moves them from the renal tubular lumen into the peritubular capillaries.

Complete the Sentences

45. microvilli
46. nephron; juxtamedullary
47. mesangial
48. renal plasma flow
49. sympathetic; vasoconstrict
50. favor; oppose
51. renalase
52. erythropoietin; erythropoiesis
53. clearance
54. increases; chronic
55. increases; catabolism

Finish the Descriptions

56. In the spinal cord, the sensory neurons activate parasympathetic motor pathways that cause the bladder muscle to contract. Inhibition of the sympathetic innervation of the internal urethral sphincter accompanies this process. Unless this reflex is inhibited voluntarily, micturition occurs.
57. Renal afferent arterioles constrict, which prevents an increase in filtration pressure. This protects the glomeruli from damage and maintains renal excretion.
58. In the blood, renin converts angiotensinogen to angiotensin I, which angiotensin-converting enzyme changes to angiotensin II, a vasoconstrictor. Angiotensin II also stimulates secretion of aldosterone from the adrenal cortex. Aldosterone circulates to the kidneys, where it increases reabsorption of sodium and water and excretion of potassium.

Teach People about Physiology

Compare your answers with these sample answers.

59. The walls of the ureters have special muscles that contract in rhythmic waves we call peristalsis. That is similar to the way that digested food moves through the intestines. Peristalsis moves the urine to the bladder regardless of body position.
60. The arterial blood that is not filtered at the glomerulus enters another capillary bed before it leaves the kidney. That capillary bed is the peritubular capillaries that surround the renal tubules; it is important in allowing the tubules to reabsorb and secrete substances to produce the proper composition of the urine. After the peritubular capillaries, the blood goes into the renal venous system and back into the systemic veins.
61. Remember that these refugees come to us with protein malnutrition. Our kidneys need urea from the normal breakdown of protein in order to concentrate the urine. If there is not enough protein in the body, there will not be enough urea, and the kidneys will not be able to do their maximal job of concentrating the urine.
62. That number is correct. We do not urinate out our body fluids because the kidney tubules that receive that filtered fluid put about 99% of the fluid back into the blood. So we only urinate out what the kidneys have selected for excretion, and we keep the rest of the fluid in our bodies.
63. The basic change is a decrease in the number of nephrons as people age. Among other changes, that decreases the ability to concentrate the urine. Thus you make a larger urine volume at night than you used to make, and you wake up to urinate. Some changes in bladder function with age may contribute to nocturia as well.

CHAPTER 30

Match the Definitions

1. C
2. A
3. D
4. B

Circle the Correct Words

5. kills
6. undergoes hypertrophy of existing glomeruli and tubules
7. calcium phosphate; uric acid
8. neurogenic bladder
9. bladder; painless
10. retrograde up the urethra; retrograde up a ureter
11. confusion
12. renal tubules; pain
13. histologic appearance
14. irreversible; chronic kidney disease

Categorize the Causes

15. Intrarenal
16. Prerenal
17. Intrarenal
18. Postrenal
19. Postrenal

Identify the Examples

20. D
21. A
22. B
23. C

Describe the Differences

24. Cystitis is inflammation of the urinary bladder, but pyelonephritis is inflammation of a kidney.
25. Azotemia is accumulation of nitrogenous wastes in the blood, manifested as elevated BUN and often creatinine as well, but uremia is a syndrome that includes azotemia and numerous other clinical manifestations such as fatigue, anemia, and pruritus.

Complete the Sentences

26. calculi; calcium
27. prostate; pelvic organs
28. carcinomas
29. interstitial
30. immune
31. diabetes
32. acute kidney injury; chronic kidney disease
33. 400

Match the Clinical Manifestations

34. D
35. F
36. A
37. C
38. B
39. G
40. E

Complete the Table

Normal Renal Function	Result of Impaired Function in the Uremic Syndrome
Excrete nitrogenous wastes	Azotemia (elevated BUN and plasma creatinine)
Excrete potassium ions	Hyperkalemia
Excrete metabolic acids	Metabolic acidosis
Excrete phosphate	Hyperphosphatemia and hypocalcemia
Activate vitamin D	Hypocalcemia, secondary hyperparathyroidism, renal osteodystrophy
Secrete erythropoietin	Anemia
Excrete sodium and water	Extracellular fluid volume excess, hypertension, potential for pulmonary edema

Teach People about Pathophysiology

Compare your answers with these sample answers.

41. Casts are little molds of the inside of the little tubes in your kidneys that help make urine. When you have a kidney infection, white blood cells go into the kidney to fight the infection. Some of them stick inside the little tubes and make these casts, which detach and go out in the urine. The casts do not injure you. They are the protective white blood cells. Having white blood cell casts in the urine is a sign that you have a kidney infection.
42. When you have a bladder infection, there is a risk for the infection going up into your kidneys. That risk increases during pregnancy because the urine tubes from the kidneys to the bladder are more relaxed during pregnancy. Chills and fever occur with a bacterial infection; if you develop a kidney infection, it likely will signal itself with chills and fever. If that happens, call the office so that the infection can be treated rapidly.
43. Yes, being tired does come from your kidney disease. You know that kidneys normally make urine. Kidneys also have another normal function: they release a hormone called erythropoietin that stimulates bone marrow to make new red blood cells. Red blood cells normally carry oxygen to all parts of your body. With your chronic kidney disease, your kidneys are not making enough of that erythropoietin hormone that stimulates red blood cell production. Without the proper signals, your bone marrow does not make enough red blood cells, and your muscles and other parts of your body do not get the oxygen you need. That makes you very tired. In addition, if the potassium is high in your blood, that can make your muscles weak, which can contribute to being tired.
44. I know it is difficult not to eat strawberries when they are in season, but there is a good reason for you to avoid them. Strawberries contain a lot of potassium. As you know, your kidneys cannot make enough urine. Normally, when we eat strawberries and other potassium-rich foods, our kidneys excrete the extra potassium in the urine, so it does not build up in the blood. Because your kidneys are not able to do that, if you eat strawberries, the potassium will build up in your blood and can cause your heart to beat irregularly or even stop. So it really is important for you not to eat a lot of strawberries.
45. Kidney damage can be in different amounts. The nephrons are the parts of your kidneys that help make urine. If you still have some functioning kidney tissue, but a lot of your nephrons are not working properly, your kidneys will lose their ability to concentrate urine. Normally, our kidneys concentrate the urine more at night, so we urinate less at night. However, you are making more urine than usual because your kidneys are not able to concentrate it. That is why you are getting up to urinate at night.
46. You do have a kidney stone. That kidney stone stuck in your ureter and the urine backed up into your kidney, stretching part of the inside of your kidney.

The enlarged kidney from accumulation of urine is called hydronephrosis.

47. His renal tubules are recovering, so he is making more urine, but he is not able to concentrate urine well because he is not fully recovered.

48. Normally, glomerular membranes have a negative charge which keeps negatively charged proteins like albumin out of the urine. In nephrotic syndrome, the glomerular membranes have lost their normal negative charges. That enables massive amounts of proteins to move into the renal tubules.

49. Stress incontinence is involuntary loss of urine control when there is more pressure in the abdomen, like when coughing or laughing. Do you know someone who has developed stress incontinence?

50. There are many causes of anemia. Heavy menstruation takes iron from our bodies, and raisins help put it back. It sounds like you did a good job with that. However, now your anemia has a different cause. Your kidneys are not stimulating your bone marrow properly, so your bone marrow is not making enough red blood cells. Raisins can put more potassium in your blood than your kidneys can handle, so you should not eat them.

51. The location of the injury determines what bladder dysfunction will occur. Lesions in the sacral area of the spinal cord or peripheral nerves that innervate the bladder cause underactive, hypotonic, or flaccid bladder function, often with loss of bladder sensation. Lesions in the brain or spinal cord above the sacral area cause loss of coordinated neuromuscular contraction and overactive or hyperreflexive bladder function.

CHAPTER 31

Match the Definitions

1. D
2. A
3. C
4. B

Circle the Correct Words

5. cystitis; decreases
6. girls
7. difficult; enuresis
8. 5
9. idiopathic; absence
10. bladder outlet

Explain the Pictures

11. In picture B, the ureter travels straight through the bladder wall, whereas in picture A, it crosses at an oblique angle.
12. Picture A
13. Vesicoureteral reflux

14. When the bladder wall contracts, the ureter continues to be patent, and urine refluxes up the ureter, flowing back into the bladder as the bladder relaxes.

15. If bacteria reach the bladder, they are less likely to be flushed out, which increases the risk for cystitis. Reflux of infected urine up the ureter to the kidney predisposes to pyelonephritis.

Describe the Differences

16. In hypospadias, the urethral meatus is located on the ventral side of the penis, but in epispadias, it is located on the dorsal side of the penis.

17. A hypoplastic kidney is small with fewer nephrons but otherwise normal, but a dysplastic kidney contains abnormal tissue.

18. Primary incontinence occurs when a child has not developed bladder control beyond the age at which bladder control usually is achieved, but secondary incontinence occurs when a child who has been dry for at least 6 months becomes incontinent again.

19. Chordee is a congenital defect in which the penis bends ventrally, but penile torsion is a congenital defect in which the penile shaft is twisted.

Complete the Sentences

20. horseshoe
21. exstrophy
22. ureteropelvic junction; hydronephrosis
23. nephroblastoma; kidney; abdomen
24. hypoalbuminemia; edema; periorbital

Teach People about Pathophysiology

Compare your answers with these sample answers.

25. Yes, that foamy urine is part of her nephrotic syndrome. Her urine is foamy because it has a lot of protein in it. Usually that protein stays in the blood, but with nephrotic syndrome, the protein barrier in the kidneys is not working, and proteins go into the urine.

26. *Poly* means "a lot" and *cystic* refers to cysts, which are little sacs that are filled with fluid in polycystic kidney disease. So polycystic kidney disease is a condition in which a lot of little sacs form in the kidneys and fill up with fluid. As more and more cysts form, they compress the normal kidney tissue, so that it cannot function.

27. Normally, the amniotic fluid surrounding the developing baby helps the lungs develop. Part of that fluid comes from the developing baby's kidneys. When the developing baby's kidneys do not form correctly, there is less of that useful amniotic fluid. Thus the lungs do not develop well.

Clinical Scenario

28. No, the strep organism did not infect Shane's kidneys. What happened is that his immune system

learned to defend against the strep organism, and after the strep was all gone, Shane's immune system attacked his kidneys and damaged them.

29. The smoky brown color is caused by hematuria; the red blood cells leak through spaces in the damaged glomeruli.

30. Shane's glomerular filtration rate decreased because of damaged glomeruli with thickened glomerular membranes. His kidneys retained sodium and water, increasing his vascular hydrostatic pressure, which promotes edema, especially in dependent areas like the ankles.

31. In acute poststreptococcal glomerulonephritis, antigen-antibody complexes form or lodge in the glomeruli, which causes inflammation and glomerular damage.

32. In Henoch-Schönlein purpura nephritis, the clinical manifestations include purpura and arthritis in addition to the renal ones.

CHAPTER 32

Match the Definitions

1. B
2. C
3. E
4. A
5. D

Circle the Correct Words

6. occurs only during fetal life; begins at puberty
7. 1 year
8. low
9. estradiol
10. LH and FSH; anterior; GnRH
11. progesterone
12. low; high

Order the Steps

13. B, D, C, A, E

Explain the Pictures

14. Y; testes
15. ovaries; wolffian (mesonephric)
16. The müllerian ducts join and become the uterus, fallopian tubes, cervix, and upper two thirds of the vagina.
17. male; female
18. Both Bartholin and Cowper glands secrete substances that enhance the motility and viability of sperm.
19. A = menstruation; B = proliferative phase; C = secretory phase; D = ischemic phase; E = menstruation
20. Secretory phase
21. Progesterone
22. Estrogen
23. Ovulation

Describe the Differences

24. Puberty is the onset of sexual maturation, but adolescence is the stage of human development between childhood and adulthood and includes social, psychological, and biological changes.

25. Menarche is the beginning of menstruation, but menopause is the cessation of menstruation.

Complete the Sentences

26. 23
27. clitoris
28. endometrium; basal
29. fundus
30. corpus luteum
31. androgens (or androstenedione); testosterone
32. luteal
33. fallopian tube

Teach People about Physiology

Compare your answers with these sample answers.

34. As women age, the character of the vagina changes. The lining gets thinner. The secretions become fewer and less acidic, which makes a more favorable environment for microorganisms to grow and cause infection. So you are more vulnerable to infection now that you are older.

35. Yes, those fringes, or fimbriae to use their technical name, have an important purpose. See how they are near the ovary? When an ovary releases an egg, those fringes move and create a current that draws the egg into the fallopian tube so that the egg can travel down the tube toward the uterus. Do you want to know where the egg gets fertilized?

36. Yes, there is a good reason. Because of the hormonal changes during the menstrual cycle, your breasts are likely to be the fullest and most tender right before menstruation and less tender afterward. A mammogram right after your menstrual period will be more comfortable for you.

37. Heat is bad for developing sperm. That is why the testicles hang outside the body, to keep them cool so that they can make sperm. If you sit in the hot tub, you will get your testicles too hot, which can decrease your sperm count and reduce your chances of having a baby.

CHAPTER 33

Match the Definitions

1. E
2. D
3. H
4. A
5. G
6. I

7. B
8. C
9. F

Circle the Correct Words

10. luteal
11. acid
12. chronic pain of; duct
13. obesity; pelvic
14. estrogen; excessive
15. columnar; squamous
16. asymptomatic; bleeding
17. estrogen; progesterone
18. are not; fibrocystic disease
19. vaginismus

Explain the Pictures

20. In Figure A (ductal carcinoma in situ), the proliferating cells have not crossed the basement membrane, but in Figure B (advanced breast cancer), they have crossed it and invaded other breast tissues.
21. No, DCIS does not always progress to invasive cancer.
22. Figure B
23. Painless
24. Within the same tumor, breast cancer often is heterogeneous. Tumors evolve. The cancer cells can vary in their multiple mutations; the tumor also includes macrophages and fibroblasts that are recruited to the tumor, become part of its microenvironment, and drive development of heterogeneity of the cancer cells.

Categorize the Risk Factors

25. Familial
26. Environmental
27. Reproductive (also could be considered hormonal)
28. Environmental
29. Hormonal
30. Environmental
31. Environmental
32. Hormonal
33. Familial

Describe the Differences

34. Primary dysmenorrhea is associated with excessive endometrial prostaglandins in ovulatory cycles, in the absence of pelvic disease, but secondary dysmenorrhea is associated with pelvic disease.
35. Primary amenorrhea is the absence of menstruation by a specific age, but secondary amenorrhea is the absence of menstruation for a time equivalent to more than three cycles in women who have previously menstruated.
36. Menorrhagia is excessive and prolonged menstrual bleeding, but metrorrhagia is uterine bleeding between menstrual cycles.

37. Vaginitis is vaginal inflammation with presence of white blood cells on saline wet prep examination, but vaginosis is vaginal inflammation without white blood cells.
38. Endometriosis is the presence of functioning endometrial tissue outside the uterus, but adenomyosis is the presence of endometrial glands surrounded by benign endometrial stroma within the uterine myometrium.

Complete the Sentences

39. 13
40. 6; 7; 9
41. endometriosis
42. hypothalamus; anterior; FSH; estrogen
43. salpingitis; pelvic inflammatory
44. dermoid
45. human papilloma; cervical
46. galactorrhea; prolactin; pituitary

Teach People about Pathophysiology

Compare your answers with these sample answers.

47. Gonorrhea can lead to pelvic inflammatory disease and scar the fallopian tubes.
48. With fibrocystic breast disease, there is extra connective tissue that is like scar tissue, and little fluid-filled sacs form in the breast. You are correct that it is not cancer.
49. Normally, friendly bacteria live in the vagina; they keep the yeast organisms from multiplying. Antibiotics get rid of the bacteria that cause a bladder infection, but they also get rid of the friendly bacteria in the vagina. That provides an opportunity for the yeast to grow.
50. A follicular cyst occurs when the dominant follicle fails to rupture or one or more of the nondominant follicles fail to regress. The causes are not well understood but most likely result from altered levels of the hormones involved in the ovarian cycle.
51. Some of the cells that normally are part of the lining of the uterus have migrated into places in your body where they do not belong. That tissue responds to your hormonal cycles and bleeds when you are menstruating. Because the blood is trapped inside your body, it causes inflammation and pain.
52. Women who have uterine cancer often develop vaginal bleeding like you did, and their cancer gets diagnosed and treated in the early stages. However, people who have ovarian cancer usually do not have symptoms that can call attention to the cancer, so their cancer gets diagnosed and treated late, sometimes after it has spread to other organs.

Clinical Scenarios

53. The most common infecting organisms in PID are bacteria; bacterial infections usually cause fever.

54. PID includes infection of the uterus, fallopian tubes, and ovaries.
55. Dyspareunia
56. Dyschezia
57. Dyspareunia and dyschezia occur with PID because Jodie has widespread inflammation in her pelvic organs, which sensitizes pain receptors.
58. Jodie has already indicated that she experiences increased pain when she jumps or tries to walk briskly.
59. Potential complications of PID that Jodie may experience in the future include infertility, ectopic pregnancy, and pelvic adhesions with chronic pelvic pain.
60. Elevated testosterone, hirsutism, and acne
61. Increased
62. Increased
63. Obesity is common with PCOS. In addition, recent weight gain tends to exacerbate the signs and symptoms.
64. Insulin helps raise free testosterone levels by stimulating androgen secretion by the ovary and reducing sex hormone–binding globulin (SHBG) in the blood. Excessive androgens affect follicular growth and contribute to anovulation; insulin affects follicular decline by suppressing apoptosis and enabling follicles, which would normally disintegrate, to survive.

CHAPTER 34

Match the Definitions

1. K
2. I
3. H
4. J
5. C
6. A
7. B
8. D
9. F
10. E
11. G

Circle the Correct Words

12. estrogen
13. rise
14. squamous cell carcinoma; adenocarcinoma
15. mumps
16. ischemia and necrosis
17. inner layers; periphery
18. by ascending the urinary tract; pyelonephritis
19. erection

Describe the Differences

20. In phimosis, the foreskin cannot be retracted over the glans penis, but in paraphimosis, the foreskin is retracted and cannot be returned to its normal position over the glans.
21. Delayed puberty comes abnormally late (no clinical signs of puberty by age 14), but precocious puberty comes abnormally early (sexual maturation before age 9).
22. Although both are scrotal masses, a varicocele consists of abnormally dilated veins within the spermatic cord, and a hydrocele is a collection of fluid within the tunica vaginalis.

Complete the Sentences

23. seminoma
24. chemical epididymitis
25. estrogens
26. erection, emission, ejaculation
27. estrogen/testosterone

Teach People about Pathophysiology

Compare your answers with these sample answers.

28. As you know, your prostate gland is enlarged. The prostate gland surrounds the urethra, the tube through which the urine flows when you empty your bladder. When your prostate gland got bigger on the outside, it also grew on the inside, squeezing your urethra, so it is narrower. It is like stepping on a garden hose and compressing it but not totally squashing it flat. Not as much water will flow through the narrow hose. With your enlarged prostate, the urine has to flow through a narrower tube, so it takes longer to empty your bladder.
29. Unlike many other cancers, many prostate cancers grow very slowly. So it actually is possible to watch them rather than do surgery to remove them.
30. No, you do not have gonorrhea. *Nongonococcal* means that some other microorganism, not the one that causes gonorrhea, caused your urethritis. It could be *Chlamydia* or another organism.
31. That procedure with the flashlight is called transillumination, and it is a standard way of diagnosing a hydrocele. The light shines through the skin differently if there is fluid inside or a solid mass. It sounds like he definitely knows how to help you.
32. Undescended testicles are associated with increased risk for testicular cancer. Testicular cancer can spread to nearby lymph nodes; he was feeling your groin lymph nodes to see if they are enlarged.

CHAPTER 35

Match the Definitions

1. C
2. D
3. E
4. A
5. B

Match the Cells

6. D
7. A
8. B
9. C
10. G
11. H
12. E
13. I
14. F

Circle the Correct Words

15. stimulate; delay
16. liver; alkaline
17. its secretion
18. immunoglobulin A
19. peristalsis
20. delay; delay
21. microvilli
22. small; initial; small
23. sterile; weeks
24. liver; bile
25. inactive; active; active
26. decrease; decrease

Categorize the Stimuli

27. Increase
28. Decrease
29. Increase
30. Increase
31. Decrease
32. Increase

Order the Steps

33. B, D, F, A, C, E

Explain the Picture

34. The liver
35. Liver lobule
36. Sinusoids
37. Branches of the hepatic portal vein and the hepatic artery
38. Central veins
39. The highly permeable endothelium that lines the sinusoids enables movement of nutrients, drugs, and other molecules into the hepatocytes, where they are metabolized.
40. The canaliculi, which empty into the bile ducts

Describe the Differences

41. The upper part of the esophagus has striated muscle, but the lower part has smooth muscle.
42. The visceral layer of the peritoneum covers the abdominal organs, but the parietal layer extends along the abdominal wall.
43. The antrum of the stomach is the lower portion, but the fundus is the upper portion.
44. A micelle is a water-soluble collection of bile salts and various forms of fat and cholesterol in the intestinal lumen, but a chylomicron is a water-soluble collection of triglycerides, cholesterol, and lipoproteins that circulate in the lymph and blood.

Match the Enzymes

45. E
46. F
47. D
48. B
49. C
50. A

Complete the Sentences

51. celiac; superior mesenteric
52. duodenum; jejunum; ileum
53. lacteal; fat (or lipid)
54. secretion; absorption
55. pyloric; Oddi
56. ileocecal; closed
57. transverse; descending; sigmoid
58. smooth; striated
59. round; falciform; abdominal
60. cholesterol; enterohepatic
61. enterokinase
62. submucosa; muscularis
63. enteric; myenteric

Teach People about Physiology

Compare your answers with these sample answers.

64. Mucus in the stomach protects the wall of the stomach from the acid and digestive enzymes that could damage it. The mucus forms a protective barrier.
65. Pepsin is sensitive to how acid its environment is. In an acid environment like the stomach, pepsin is active, but in a less acid (more alkaline) environment like the intestine, pepsin does not function any more.
66. Eating some vitamin C at the same time as the iron pill helps the iron enter the body (be absorbed) more easily. The vitamin C reduces ferric iron to ferrous iron, which is the form more easily absorbed.
67. The appendix is attached to the first portion of the large intestine. After the stomach, food travels into the small intestine and then the large intestine before the waste exits our bodies as a bowel movement. The appendix hangs off the initial part of the large intestine like a little pouch.
68. The gastrocolic reflex helps us have a bowel movement right after eating. When the stomach is stretched by food and partially digested food enters portions of the small intestine, the large intestine

starts contracting mor? and moves its contents onward to become a bowel movement.

69. Bile is important and useful. It helps process dietary fats in the intestine so that the animal or the person gets the benefit from eating the fats. Bile is made by the liver and stored in the gallbladder until it goes into the intestines when the animal or person eats fats.

CHAPTER 36 _____

Match the Definitions

1. D
2. F
3. B
4. J
5. A
6. H
7. C
8. G
9. I
10. E

Circle the Correct Words

11. decreased; lower; cough
12. sliding; is
13. vomiting; constipation
14. digestive enzymes; necrotic; peritonitis
15. hypothalamus; peripheral; body fat mass
16. Visceral; leptin; adiponectin
17. intrahepatic; posthepatic
18. hypertension; vasodilation; bacterial
19. yellow; sclera of the eye

Categorize the Clinical Manifestations

20. Portal hypertension
21. Hepatocyte dysfunction
22. Hepatocyte dysfunction
23. Portal hypertension
24. Portal hypertension
25. Portal hypertension
26. Hepatocyte dysfunction

Order the Steps

27. D, B, F, A, E, C, G

Characterize the Types of Hepatitis

Describe the Differences

28. GERD (gastroesophageal reflux disease) is reflux of acid and pepsin from the stomach to the esophagus that causes esophagitis, but NERD (nonerosive reflux disease) involves similar symptoms with no visible sign of esophagitis.
29. Type A chronic gastritis is caused by autoimmune damage primarily in the gastric fundus, but type B chronic gastritis is caused by nonimmune mechanisms such as *H. pylori*, chronic use of alcohol, and nonsteroidal anti-inflammatory drugs and occurs primarily in the gastric antrum.
30. Maldigestion is failure of the chemical processes of breaking down (digesting) nutrients that take place in the intestinal lumen or at the brush border of the intestinal mucosa of the small intestine, but malabsorption is the failure of the intestinal mucosa to transport the digested nutrients into the blood or lymph.
31. Orexigenic neurons promote eating, but anorexigenic neurons inhibit eating.
32. In short-term starvation, the body responds with glycogenolysis and gluconeogenesis with only a small amount of protein catabolism, but in long-term starvation, the body responds with lipolysis and eventually proteolysis that can cause death.
33. In alcoholic cirrhosis, the damage begins with the hepatocytes, but in biliary cirrhosis, the damage begins in the bile canaliculi and bile ducts.

Match the Disorders

34. B
35. G
36. D
37. F
38. A
39. I
40. E
41. C
42. J
43. H

Complete the Sentences

44. achalasia
45. hiatal hernia
46. alkalosis; acidosis
47. days

Characteristic	Hepatitis A Infection	Hepatitis B Infection	Hepatitis C Infection	Hepatitis D Infection	Hepatitis E Infection
Route of transmission	Fecal-oral, parenteral, sexual	Parenteral, sexual, across placenta	Parenteral, sexual, across placenta	Parenteral (?), fecal-oral, sexual	Fecal-oral
Acute or chronic?	Acute	Acute or chronic	Acute or chronic	Chronic	Acute
Carrier state	No	Yes	Yes	Yes	No

48. peptic; *pylori*
49. fat; lipase
50. mucosa; colon
51. periumbilical; right lower
52. 30; exceeds
53. adipokines; macrophages
54. D
55. icteric; recovery
56. cystic; cholesterol
57. lipase; alcohol
58. alcohol; obesity; cirrhosis

Complete the Chart

Characteristics	Crohn Disease	Ulcerative Colitis
Family history	More common	Less common
Location of lesions	Entire GI tract, with small and large intestines most common, skip lesions	Rectum and colon, continuous lesions
Nature of lesions	Involve entire thickness of intestinal wall	Involve mucosal layer only
Fistulas and abscesses	Common	Rare
Narrowed lumen, possible obstruction	Common	Rare
Recurrent episodes of diarrhea	Common	Common
Blood in stools	Less common	Common
Clinical course	Remissions and exacerbations	Remissions and exacerbations

Match the Risk Factors

59. D
60. A
61. B
62. C

Teach People about Pathophysiology

Compare your answers with these sample answers.

63. With alcoholic hepatitis, the liver is inflamed, and there are necrotic cells because of the alcohol damage, so the person has signs and symptoms of acute inflammation and liver dysfunction. The liver often regenerates and recovers from hepatitis if the person stops drinking. With alcoholic cirrhosis, alcohol damage triggers overgrowth of connective tissue (fibrosis) that distorts the liver. Although hepatocytes regenerate, they are not connected properly to blood vessels or bile ducts, so the person has hepatocyte dysfunction. In addition, liver fibrosis obstructs the portal vessels that flow into the liver, causing pressure to rise in the portal system. Portal hypertension and hepatocyte dysfunction cause the signs and symptoms of cirrhosis. Cirrhosis usually is considered to be irreversible.

64. Barrett esophagus occurs in people who have heartburn with GERD, but it is not the same as heartburn. The term describes physical changes that have occurred in the esophagus when there has been a lot of acid reflux. Normal esophagus cells do not live well in a location where there is a lot of acid and other substances from the stomach. If acid reflux occurs again and again, the body replaces the normal esophagus cells with other types of normal cells that can endure the acid. Barrett esophagus is not cancer, but it is a warning sign that a portion of the esophagus is at risk for cancer.

65. Some of the enzymes that the pancreas normally makes are inactive enzymes, and they are not activated until they reach the intestines where they digest food. However, in pancreatitis, those enzymes become activated inside the pancreas, so they start digesting the pancreas and cause damage and pain.

66. You both definitely have a lot of stress right now. Your wife is unconscious, but her body is experiencing a lot of physical stress that causes some physiologic changes. Stress ulcers are multiple little areas of injury in the lining of the stomach that occur in people who have injuries serious enough that they need to be in the ICU. Stress ulcers do not cause any pain, although they can bleed. We are taking the best care possible of your wife. Now let us talk about your stress. What ways do you have of managing it?

67. Some bile and secretions from your pancreas are going backward into your stomach remnant, where they are not supposed to go. They contain substances that damage the inside wall of your stomach remnant.

68. A healthy liver removes potentially harmful substances from the blood and changes them chemically so they are not harmful. When the liver does not work well, potentially harmful substances build up in the blood and can circulate to the brain. They change how the brain works, which causes the confusion and drowsiness you see in your husband.

69. The hepatocytes in a well-functioning liver synthesize albumin and put it into the blood. In cirrhosis, many of the hepatocytes have been destroyed or are not working well, so the liver is not able to synthesize enough albumin to keep the blood levels normal.

292

Clinical Scenario

70. T; microflora
71. The physician needed to check for appendicitis as a possible cause of Ms. Hawk's abdominal pain.
72. Active episodes of ulcerative colitis often involve bloody diarrhea; she already has developed iron deficiency anemia from blood loss.
73. Several gastrointestinal disorders cause diarrhea and crampy abdominal pain, including ulcerative colitis and Crohn disease. A colonoscopy provides a view of the colonic mucosa that assists with the diagnosis.
74. Although a positive family history is less common with ulcerative colitis than with Crohn disease, ulcerative colitis does have a genetic component that sets the stage for abnormal immune response that damages the bowel mucosa.
75. People who have ulcerative colitis have high risk for developing colon cancer, especially if they have had the condition for numerous years. It is important to detect colon cancer in the early stages before it metastasizes so that it can be treated successfully. Ms. Hawk's mother had surgery for colon cancer.
76. She needs to replace the salt and water that are being lost in the diarrhea. If she has continued diarrhea and does not replace the fluid and salt, she will develop clinical dehydration, the combination of extracellular fluid volume deficit and hypernatremia.

CHAPTER 37

Match the Definitions

1. D
2. C
3. A
4. B

Circle the Correct Words

5. other anomalies
6. cleft; feeding
7. B and C; no
8. volvulus
9. dilation; collapse
10. third
11. cystic fibrosis
12. acute diarrhea

Categorize the Conditions

13. Congenital
14. Congenital
15. Acquired
16. Congenital
17. Congenital
18. Acquired
19. Acquired
20. Congenital
21. Acquired
22. Acquired

Order the Steps

23. C, A, D, B

Explain the Picture

24. Esophageal atresia
25. Excessive amount of amniotic fluid is associated with esophageal atresia because normally the fetus swallows amniotic fluid that then absorbs into the placental circulation. Because the esophagus is a blind pouch, this process cannot occur, and the volume of amniotic fluid increases.
26. Tracheoesophageal fistula
27. Air will enter the stomach, distending it; gastric secretions will regurgitate into the trachea and enter the lungs, causing inflammation by damaging lung tissue.

Describe the Differences

28. Marasmus is severe acute malnutrition caused by deficiency of all nutrients, but kwashiorkor is severe acute malnutrition caused by deficiency of protein.
29. Physiologic jaundice occurs in the first week after birth and is not associated with underlying disease, but pathologic jaundice has higher bilirubin levels and is associated with disease.

Match the Risk Factors

30. C
31. A
32. D
33. B

Complete the Sentences

34. recessive; copper; liver
35. bile; jaundice
36. celiac; T; epithelium
37. fat
38. fat; muscle
39. kernicterus
40. necrotizing enterocolitis; bowel; death
41. pancreatic; mucus; sweat

Match the Signs and Symptoms

42. C
43. D
44. A
45. E
46. B

Teach People about Pathophysiology

Compare your answers with these sample answers.

47. Because they do not eat until after they are born, new-born babies normally have meconium in their intestines. Normal meconium moves easily through the intestines and comes out when the bowels move. The usual cause of having thick meconium like your baby does is lack of some digestive enzymes. That is why they are doing some tests, to determine what the problem is. Meanwhile, the enema should help to soften the thick meconium so it will move out as it should.

48. That little pouch on Travis's intestine has some cells inside it that normally belong in the stomach. Those cells are making acid and strong digestive enzymes like they are supposed to do in the stomach; however, the acid and enzymes are in the little intestinal pouch where they damage the pouch wall. That damage makes an ulcer, which is an open sore that can bleed. That is why Travis was bleeding into his intestine and you saw the blood in his diaper.

49. The word *aganglionic* explains the problem with Diego's bowel. Normally there are collections of nerve cells called ganglia in the wall of the bowel. The nerves normally make the bowel muscles contract and move the bowel contents. Diego does not have all of the normal ganglia in a portion of his bowel wall, so the bowel contents do not move through it. They collect behind that part of his bowel and distend it, making it big.

50. When the bowel contents stop moving, they get hard and stuck. We call that impacted. The hard mass does not move, but liquid can go around it, so that is why Diego had some watery diarrhea.

51. Normally, the small intestine has little projections, like tiny fingers, that are called villi. They stick into the liquid contents of the intestine and move the nutrients into the body. When the villi are flattened, as happened to Nina, there is less chance to take the nutrients into the body. Nina needs nutrients from her food so she can grow. As long as you avoid gluten in her diet, her intestine will have a chance to repair itself and function more normally again.

CHAPTER 38

Match the Definitions

1. F
2. E
3. A
4. B
5. D
6. C

Match the Cell Functions

7. E
8. D
9. F
10. G
11. B
12. C
13. A

Circle the Correct Words

14. cancellous
15. canaliculi; lacunae
16. endurance; prevent fatigue; provide precision of movement
17. sarcoplasmic reticulum membranes; calcium
18. tension; length; tension

Categorize the Substances

19. Inhibits
20. Facilitates
21. Facilitates
22. Facilitates
23. Inhibits
24. Facilitates

Order the Steps

25. C, A, B, D
26. E, B, A, C, D
27. E, C, A, G, B, D, F, H

Explain the Pictures

28. articular; type II collagen
29. cancellous (spongy); Red marrow
30. marrow; Yellow marrow (fatty tissue)
31. compact; cortical
32. periosteum; Connective
33. diaphysis
34. B and D
35. B
36. D
37. I band
38. A band
39. I band

Describe the Differences

40. Compact bone is solid, extremely strong, and highly organized, with its basic structural unit being the haversian system, but cancellous bone is less complex and forms an irregular meshwork composed of trabeculae that branch and unite with one another.
41. A diarthrosis is a freely movable joint, but a synarthrosis is an immovable joint, and an amphiarthrosis is a slightly movable joint.
42. Osteoid is the matrix of bone that is not yet mineralized, but bone is the fully mineralized structure.
43. A synovial joint is connected by a fibrous joint capsule that contains a fluid-filled space, but a symphysis is a cartilaginous joint in which bones are united by a pad of fibrocartilage, such as the intervertebral disks.

Complete the Sentences

44. bone morphogenic; osteoblasts
45. collagen
46. subchondral; tidemark
47. fascia
48. motor unit
49. debt; lactic
50. sarcopenia

Compare and Contrast the Muscle Fibers

Characteristic	Type I Fibers	Type II Fibers
Speed of Contraction	Slow	Fast
Intensity of Contraction	Low	High
Type of Metabolism	Oxidative	Glycolysis
Number of Mitochondria	Many	Few
Amount of Myoglobin	High	Low
Color	Red	White
Capillary Supply	Profuse	Intermediate to sparse

Teach People about Physiology

Compare your answers with these sample answers.

51. Osteocytes are osteoblasts that are terminally differentiated; in other words, they are fully matured and no longer build bone. They are located in small spaces in the bones and communicate with both osteoblasts and osteoclasts about when and where to form and resorb bone as well as other functions that keep bone functional.

52. The normal fluid in your knee joint, called synovial fluid, supplies nourishment to the cartilage. Synovial fluid is filtered from the blood, so it contains the nourishment your cartilage needs.

53. There is no difference; those terms refer to the same muscles. The term *striated* refers to the striped pattern that people see when they look at skeletal muscle with a microscope.

54. You ask an important question! Muscles need increased intracellular calcium to contract, and then they need less calcium so they can relax. The sarcotubular system releases calcium for muscle contraction and then takes it up and stores the calcium during muscle relaxation.

55. The term *lean body mass* is another way of saying "muscle mass." So they are talking about bulking up their muscles.

56. Muscles take in creatine from the blood. They change some of it into phosphocreatine, which provides energy for muscle contraction. Our bodies normally make creatine, so you already have some creatine in your blood.

CHAPTER 39

Match the Definitions

1. B
2. E
3. F
4. A
5. C
6. D

Circle the Correct Words

7. substantial
8. sprain; strain
9. weeks
10. epicondylopathy
11. venous; pain
12. skeletal muscle; dark; creatine kinase; kidneys
13. bacteria; sequestrum
14. autoimmune; formation; destruction
15. break down; lysosomes
16. alcohol

Categorize the Characteristics

17. Osteoarthritis
18. Rheumatoid arthritis
19. Rheumatoid arthritis
20. Osteoarthritis
21. Rheumatoid arthritis
22. Rheumatoid arthritis
23. Rheumatoid arthritis
24. Osteoarthritis
25. Osteoarthritis
26. Rheumatoid arthritis

Order the Steps

27. A, D, G, E, F, C, B

Explain the Pictures

28. Ulnar drift
29. Rheumatoid arthritis
30. With loss of joint mobility, the person uses the hands less, and muscles surrounding the joints atrophy.
31. In rheumatoid arthritis, the joints swell initially because of synovitis, which is inflammation of the synovial membrane caused by autoimmune processes. The inflammation can spread to other joint structures.
32. Because rheumatoid arthritis is an autoimmune disease, the autoantibodies, autoreactive T lymphocytes, and other immune cells can cause damage and inflammation anywhere in the body that the autoantigens are located.
33. Osteoarthritis
34. Bouchard
35. Heberden
36. The primary cause is osteophytes (bone spurs) that develop around the margins of the joint.

37. Matrix metalloproteinases are elevated in osteoarthritis and are major contributors to the destruction of articular cartilage.

Match the Fractures

38. D
39. F
40. A
41. E
42. L
43. I
44. K
45. J
46. G
47. B
48. H
49. C

Describe the Differences

50. Delayed union is the healing together of fractured bone fragments that takes longer than usual after a fracture, but malunion is healing of a fracture with the bone in an incorrect anatomic position.
51. Dislocation is temporary displacement of a bone from its normal position in a joint, but subluxation is partial dislocation, so contact between the two joint surfaces is only partially lost.

Match the Pathophysiologies

52. D
53. F
54. E
55. A
56. B
57. C

Complete the Sentences

58. reduction; internal fixation
59. heterotopic ossification
60. skull; brain
61. metastatic; osteosarcoma
62. ground substance
63. tophi; stones
64. weakness; fatigue
65. contracture
66. spindles
67. unrestful; tender
68. disuse
69. relaxation; contraction

Match the Tumor Characteristics

70. D
71. C
72. B
73. E
74. A

Teach People about Pathophysiology

Compare your answers with these sample answers.

75. No, *compound* does not mean infected. It means that there is an open connection between the broken bone and the external environment. That exposes your bone to microorganisms that are on your skin and outside your body, which is why your doctor is concerned about infection. However, the term *compound* simply means that the skin is broken with a wound that leads to the fracture site.
76. The sore on your ankle is infected with bacteria. It is likely that some bacteria moved inward from your sore and spread directly to your bone, where they made a new infection.
77. I know you are concerned about money for food for your family. Let me tell you something important about your leg bone. When bone is healing, it lays down soft fibers around the break, and then later it makes bone in that location. That takes time. You need the cast to stabilize the two ends of the bone together so that the repair will be solid. If we take off the cast too early, the repair is not completed, and the bone could collapse or break again where it was broken. I would like to call a social worker who can help you with resources for your family while you cannot work. Would you like to talk with her?
78. Those nodes on your knuckles are part of the osteoarthritis. They are bone spurs. Osteoarthritis involves thinning and loss of cartilage in joints, but it also involves excess bone growth in some locations that makes bony bumps. The technical name for those bony bumps is osteophytes, but most people just call them bone spurs.
79. They are looking for particular substance, an enzyme called alkaline phosphatase, that certain types of bone cancers release into the blood. Knowing the amount of that substance in your blood will help them monitor the situation in your bones.

Clinical Scenario

80. Bone mass is decreased in osteopenia, but it is severely decreased in osteoporosis.
81. In osteoporosis, bone resorption occurs faster than bone formation.
82. Kyphosis in osteoporosis is caused by vertebral compression fractures.
83. Around age 30
84. It decreases.
85. In the first few years after menopause, bone mineral density decreases quite rapidly, and then it has a more gradual decline.
86. Estrogen normally stimulates production of osteoprotegerin (a protective factor) and decreases the production of RANKL (a factor that stimulates osteoclasts). Estrogen also exerts antiapoptotic effects on osteoblasts and proapoptotic effects on

osteoclasts. With less estrogen effect after menopause, osteoclast activity increases.

87. Regular, moderate weight-bearing exercise can slow down bone loss in osteoporosis. It also increases muscle strength, thus reducing her risk for falls.

CHAPTER 40

Match the Definitions

1. D
2. ᴄ
3. B
4. A

Circle the Correct Words

5. ends; midshaft
6. almost always
7. Septic arthritis; joint; joints
8. girls
9. head of the femur
10. tibial tubercle

Describe the Differences

11. Osteosarcoma is a malignant bone tumor, but osteochondroma is a benign bone tumor.
12. Osteomyelitis is bacterial infection of bone and bone marrow, but septic arthritis is bacterial infection within a joint.
13. Septic arthritis is bacterial infection within a joint, but juvenile idiopathic arthritis is an autoimmune disease that causes inflammation of joints, mostly the large joints.

Complete the Sentences

14. asymmetric
15. structural
16. osteochondroses
17. Ewing; pain
18. Still

Teach People about Pathophysiology

Compare your answers with these sample answers.

19. Osteogenesis imperfecta is a genetic disease involving defective collagen synthesis, which causes bones to break very easily. That is why it is called "brittle bone disease."
20. Your tibia was growing rapidly, but there was not enough blood supply to part of it, so that part of the bone died. Often the bone will grow back when a person rests for several weeks. You really need to rest your knee until the doctor says you can start using it again.
21. Children who are not yet walking and present with a long bone fracture have a greater than 75% chance of that fracture being caused by child abuse. Tibial fractures are common in such cases. When child abuse is

suspected, radiographs must be taken to evaluate for head trauma, other fractures, and fractures in different stages of healing.

22. An infant's bone has blood vessels that perforate the growth plate; that makes it easy for bacteria that have infected a bone to reach the joint. In older children, the arterioles end beneath the epiphyseal plate.

Clinical Scenario

23. Duchenne muscular dystrophy is inherited as an X-linked recessive condition or occurs from a sporadic mutation that silences the dystrophin gene on the short arm of the X chromosome.
24. Normally, the protein dystrophin helps anchor the actin cytoskeleton of skeletal muscle fibers to the basement membrane so that the fibers do not become damaged by the repeated stress of contraction.
25. Tommy's lower extremity and lower back muscles are weak. When he gets up from the floor, he pushes up with his hands and then uses his hands to climb up his legs until he is upright. That is the Gower sign.
26. Tommy's "waddling" gait arises from muscle weakness in his pelvic girdle. He tends to walk on his toes because of weakness of his anterior tibial and peroneal muscles.
27. CPK and the other enzymes normally are inside muscle fibers. When muscle fibers die in Duchenne muscular dystrophy, they spill their contents into the interstitial area, and these enzymes leak into the blood.
28. Tommy's calf muscles enlarged because fat and connective tissue have accumulated within them as his muscle fibers die. Because his muscles are degenerating, his calves are weak, even though they are enlarged.
29. Duchenne muscular dystrophy is a progressive degenerative disease. The shoulder girdle muscles will become involved, and he will have increasing disability. Most people who have the disease die in their mid-20s from respiratory infection and respiratory muscle weakness, although treatment continues to extend life for some.

CHAPTER 41

Match the Definitions

1. C
2. G
3. I
4. F
5. H
6. A
7. B
8. J
9. E
10. D

Circle the Correct Words

11. dermis
12. dermis
13. sympathetic; dermal
14. thinner; less; fewer
15. is not
16. virus; herald patch
17. skin; women
18. edema; inflammation
19. bacterium; tick
20. central; frontotemporal

Categorize the Disorders

21. Bacterial infection
22. Fungal infection
23. Autoimmune
24. Bacterial infection
25. Fungal infection
26. Autoimmune
27. Fungal infection
28. Autoimmune
29. Autoimmune
30. Autoimmune

Order the Layers and Note Their Functions

Latin Name of Epidermal Layer	Function of Epidermal Layer
Stratum corneum	Barrier of dead keratinocytes that protects against microorganisms and excessive water loss
Stratum granulosum	Enables keratinocytes to form granules of proteins that protect against water loss
Stratum spinosum	Enables keratinocytes to enlarge and move upward
Stratum basale (or stratum germinativum)	Formation of new keratinocytes

Explain the Pictures

31. Raised? Yes; Extends into dermis? Yes; Lesion: Cyst
32. Raised? Yes; Extends into dermis? No; Lesion: Vesicle
33. Raised? Yes; Extends into dermis? No; Lesion: Wheal
34. Raised? Yes; Extends into dermis? Yes; Lesion: Papule
35. Raised? No; Extends into dermis? No; Lesion: Macule
36. The lesion would need to be larger; a bulla is a vesicle with a diameter larger than 1 cm.

37. The lesion would need to be larger; a patch is a macule with a diameter larger than 1 cm.
38. 33
39. 32

Describe the Differences

40. A furuncle is an infection of a hair follicle that extends to the surrounding tissue, but a carbuncle is a collection of infected hair follicles that forms a draining abscess.
41. Apocrine sweat glands are fewer in number, have little known function, and are located in the axillae, scalp, face, abdomen, and genital areas, but eccrine sweat glands are more abundant, have thermoregulatory function, and are distributed over the body, with the greatest numbers in the palms of the hands, soles of the feet, and forehead.
42. A keloid is an elevated scar that extends beyond the border of the injury, but a hypertrophic scar is an elevated scar that stays within the border of the injury.
43. Acne vulgaris is the typical acne that is common in adolescence, but acne rosacea is a chronic, readily exacerbated, inflammatory skin disease that develops primarily in middle age.

Match the Functions

44. C
45. D
46. A
47. E
48. B

Complete the Sentences

49. sun; Kaposi sarcoma
50. dermatitis
51. contact; IV; delayed (or T cell mediated)
52. stasis; seborrheic
53. keratinocytes; exacerbations (or flare-ups)
54. pruritus (itching)
55. rhinophyma
56. pemphigus; autoantibodies
57. gastrointestinal tract
58. simplex; HSV-1; HSV-2
59. human papilloma; cancer

Match the Tumors

60. H
61. E
62. A
63. F
64. G
65. B
66. D
67. C

Teach People about Pathophysiology

Compare your answers with these sample answers.

68. Cells called melanocytes live in the skin where hair is formed. They make the pigments that color our hair. As we age, we have fewer of these pigment-creating cells, so our hair gets white.
69. Psoriasis is not a fungus infection. It is not an infection at all, and it is not contagious. Those silvery scaly patches on your skin are caused by excessive growth of skin cells, probably involving signals from immune cells. You can go ahead and hug your son because he will not get psoriasis from your touch.
70. We need a good flow of blood to keep our skin and the tissues beneath it healthy. Pressure ulcers develop when skin and the area beneath it do not get enough blood flow because the pressure of the body flattens the blood vessels. Without proper blood flow, the tissue dies, and an open sore develops. That happens especially over bony areas like the heels and the sacrum (the bone right above the buttocks).
71. There is no difference. *Wheals* is the technical word for a raised area of the skin that looks like hives or mosquito bites. You are correct in calling them hives. Did they tell you to stop taking the penicillin?
72. I think there is another reason that your aunt does not smile at you. Scleroderma makes the skin of the face very hard and tight, like a stiff hard plastic mask. That makes it very difficult for people to smile or move their faces when they talk. Let's find a way for you to visit with your aunt and see what she really feels.

Clinical Scenario

73. Herpes zoster
74. Varicella-zoster virus
75. It was not her first exposure to the virus. The first exposure causes chickenpox. The virus then ascends to a dorsal root ganglion, where it is dormant until it is reactivated.
76. The shingles lesions follow the distribution of the sensory nerve that the virus has infected. The virus would need to be present in both dorsal root ganglia in that dermatome to cross the midline.
77. Mrs. Maxwell is experiencing multiple stressors and therefore probably is somewhat immunosuppressed. The virus often reactivates when an individual becomes immunosuppressed.
78. Postherpetic neuralgia

CHAPTER 42

Match the Definitions

1. C
2. A
3. D
4. B

Circle the Correct Words

5. skin; immune
6. highly; staphylococci; vesicles; crust
7. circulates to
8. exanthema subitum; nonpruritic; after; infants
9. grow; shrink
10. do not

Categorize the Infections

11. Fungal
12. Bacterial
13. Fungal
14. Viral
15. Viral
16. Fungal
17. Viral
18. Viral

Explain the Picture

19. Sebum (sebaceous gland secretions)
20. Adolescents and young adults (ages 12-25)
21. Comedones (or comedos, but comedones is the technical word)
22. A whitehead
23. Hormone: androgens; bacterium: *Propionibacterium acnes*

Describe the Differences

24. Atopic dermatitis is associated with a history of allergy and an impaired epidermal barrier to allergens, but diaper dermatitis is an irritant contact dermatitis initiated by prolonged exposure to urine and feces.
25. Rubeola is measles, but rubella is German measles, a milder viral disease.
26. Variola is smallpox, but varicella is chickenpox.
27. A strawberry hemangioma is superficial, but a cavernous hemangioma is deeper.

Complete the Sentences

28. IgE; asthma
29. tinea corporis; puppies
30. proteases
31. herpes zoster; shingles
32. veins; arteries
33. bedbugs; lice; nits
34. prickly heat; sweating
35. neonatorum; weeks

Match the Clinical Manifestations

36. D
37. A
38. F
39. E
40. B
41. C

Teach People about Pathophysiology

Compare your answers with these sample answers.

42. Impetigo is quite different from chickenpox. A virus causes chickenpox, but impetigo is a bacterial infection of the skin.
43. In chickenpox (varicella), the rash begins as pruritic macules that soon become vesicles, burst, and scab over. Often, all three forms of the lesions are visible at the same time. With measles (rubeola), the rash remains macular, usually is not pruritic, and is preceded by fever. Characteristically, chickenpox rash begins on the trunk, and measles rash begins on the face. They both spread to the extremities.
44. Although rubella is a mild illness, if a pregnant woman gets rubella early in pregnancy, it causes the developing baby to have serious birth defects or even die before birth.
45. When the nurse practitioner looked in Donny's mouth, she probably saw some white spots surrounded by red rings called Koplik spots that are characteristic of measles. Along with his fever and other symptoms, Donny had a classic case of measles right before the rash appears.

Clinical Scenario

46. The linear lesions are burrows made by the scabies mite in which it lays eggs.
47. The itching probably is due to immune system sensitization to the larval stage of the scabies mite.
48. The major complication is secondary infection of the lesions damaged further by scratching.
49. Scabies is transmitted by direct contact and also through mites or eggs living on clothing or bed linen that was contaminated recently.
50. Flea bites are very different from the scabies that Angie has. Instead of the lines that you see with scabies, flea bites tend to occur in clusters. The bites are raised and have a small red puncture in the middle.